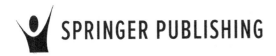
SPRINGER PUBLISHING

GET THE MOST FROM YOUR BOOK

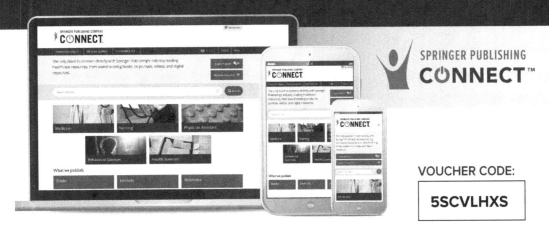

VOUCHER CODE:

5SCVLHXS

Online Access

Your print purchase of *Literature Review and Synthesis* includes **online access via Springer Publishing Connect**™ to increase accessibility, portability, and searchability.

Insert the code at https://connect.springerpub.com/content/book/978-0-8261-5214-5 today!

Having trouble? Contact our customer service department at cs@springerpub.com

Instructor Resource Access for Adopters

Let us do some of the heavy lifting to create an engaging classroom experience with a variety of instructor resources included in most textbooks SUCH AS:

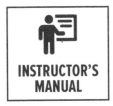

INSTRUCTOR'S MANUAL

POWERPOINTS

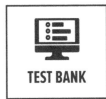

TEST BANK

Visit **https://connect.springerpub.com/** and look for the **"Show Supplementary"** button on your **book homepage** to see what is available to instructors! First time using Springer Publishing Connect?

Email **textbook@springerpub.com** to create an account and start unlocking valuable resources.

Literature Review
and Synthesis

Susan W. Buchholz, PhD, RN, ANP-BC, FAANP, FAAN, is a professor and associate dean for research at Michigan State University College of Nursing. Dr. Buchholz is funded by the National Institutes of Health National Institute of Nursing Research. Her research focuses on developing interventions for women that encourage them to lead healthier lives through small changes that make a big difference in health outcomes. In her research, she uses innovative mHealth strategies to promote physical activity. She developed a graduate level course on literature synthesis approaches that teaches nursing and other healthcare professional students how to complete an exemplary literature review and synthesis, appropriate to their own unique questions and topics. She has conducted and published quantitative and qualitative research, including systematic, integrative, and umbrella reviews. As an adult nurse practitioner faculty member, she is committed to high-quality nurse practitioner education and is currently president-elect of the National Organization of Nurse Practitioner Faculties Board. She is a fellow in the American Academy of Nursing and the American Association of Nurse Practitioners. Dr. Buchholz also served as the chair of the inaugural American Association of Nurse Practitioners Nursing Research Committee. She appreciates each day of life and is thankful for the opportunity to work with people who are committed to improving health!

Kirsten A. Dickins, PhD, AM, MSN, FNP-C, is the inaugural Connell Postdoctoral Fellow in Nursing Research at the Yvonne L. Munn Center for Nursing Research at Massachusetts General Hospital. Her research exists at the intersection of community-engaged mixed-methods approaches, health equity–focused research, aging studies, and women's health. She seeks to elucidate and address the contributors to physical, behavioral, and social health inequities through population-tailored approaches. Leveraging the voices of participants and clinicians in conjunction with clinical and public health data, her overarching research goal is to design and implement interventions that optimize primary healthcare engagements that address preventable health inequities faced by socio-structurally marginalized populations. She works as a family nurse practitioner, with a commitment to community-centered outreach models of primary care that extend beyond hospital and clinic walls. She is grateful to partake in efforts that aim toward equitable promotion of individual, community, and public health and well-being.

Literature Review and Synthesis

A Guide for Nurses and Other
Healthcare Professionals

Susan W. Buchholz, PhD, RN, ANP-BC, FAANP, FAAN

Kirsten A. Dickins, PhD, AM, MSN, FNP-C

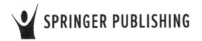 SPRINGER PUBLISHING

Springer Publishing Company, LLC
11 West 42nd Street, New York, NY 10036
www.springerpub.com
connect.springerpub.com/

Acquisitions Editor: Joseph Morita
Compositor: Transforma

ISBN: 978-0-8261-5213-8
ebook ISBN: 978-0-8261-5214-5
DOI: 10.1891/9780826152145

SUPPLEMENTS:
Instructor Materials:
Qualified instructors may request supplements by emailing textbook@springerpub.com

Instructor's Manual ISBN: 978-0-8261-6318-9

Printed by BnT

The author and the publisher of this Work have made every effort to use sources believed to be reliable to provide information that is accurate and compatible with the standards generally accepted at the time of publication. The author and publisher shall not be liable for any special, consequential, or exemplary damages resulting, in whole or in part, from the readers' use of, or reliance on, the information contained in this book. The publisher has no responsibility for the persistence or accuracy of URLs for external or third-party Internet websites referred to in this publication and does not guarantee that any content on such websites is, or will remain, accurate or appropriate.

Library of Congress Cataloging-in-Publication Data
Names: Buchholz, Susan Weber, author. | Dickins, Kirsten A., author.
Title: Literature review and synthesis : a guide for nurses and other
   healthcare professionals / Susan W. Buchholz, Kirsten A. Dickins.
Identifiers: LCCN 2021056775 | ISBN 9780826152138 (paperback) | ISBN
   9780826152145 (ebook)
Subjects: MESH: Review Literature as Topic | Systematic Reviews as Topic |
   Nurses | Delivery of Healthcare
Classification: LCC RT41 | NLM W 20.5 | DDC 610.73—dc23/eng/20211124
LC record available at https://lccn.loc.gov/2021056775

Contact sales@springerpub.com to receive discount rates on bulk purchases.

Publisher's Note: **New and used products purchased from third-party sellers are not guaranteed for quality, authenticity, or access to any included digital components.**

Printed in the United States of America.

We dedicate this book to nurses, healthcare students, and other healthcare professionals, who are advancing the science via rigorous literature review and synthesis. May your work serve to make our world a healthier place.

Contents

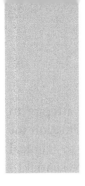

Preface

Several years ago, I was teaching a class called "Literature Synthesis Approach," which I had developed for graduate students at an academic medical center. I was fortunate to have working with me at the time a very bright doctoral student (the now Dr. Kirsten A. Dickins) who was completing her teaching practicum and had been assigned to work with me on this course. Dr. Dickins asked intriguing questions and provided scientifically based information, and together we revised and updated what was then a relatively new course. At the same time, it came to our attention that for nursing students and faculty, as well as other healthcare students and faculty who were not trained in literature review and synthesis, there was no singular manual, guide, or book that provided introductory guidance on this process. Therefore, we set about the work of strengthening materials with a multitude of resources, embedding references from the giants of the literature review world.

This book was written as a response to our experiences with the literature synthesis approach course, as well as our experiences of collaborating with others on literature reviews since that time. Literature reviews have become increasingly popular, as reviewers seek to locate and combine the multitude of scientific study results, and other sources of evidence, that abound in the fast-growing body of healthcare literature. While there exists globally an array of extraordinary literature review resources, developed by a cadre of highly trained and published scholars who are well-known to the literature review world, we found a need for a foundational literature review and synthesis book. This text, we thought, should be accessible across experience levels, straightforward to interpret, and a springboard for finding highly respected resources needed to complete exemplary literature reviews. We also came to understand the importance of involving and encouraging students early in their education to cultivate the foundational knowledge and skills of completing literature reviews and syntheses.

A central component of this book is literature synthesis. The synthesis is the "so what" of the entire literature review process—the integration of information that conveys, when taken together, what the data really mean and why the findings are important to improving health for individuals, families, communities, nations, and our global population. However, to arrive at and complete a literature synthesis, a scholar must first have the knowledge and skills to enact a series of rigorous steps that provide the scientific evidence from which the literature synthesis is created. Once the synthesis has been created, then it must be disseminated; without dissemination, this work may not reach its full potential for other healthcare professionals and policy makers whose decisions might be informed by this work.

This book is written to be used by healthcare undergraduate and graduate students, as well as nurses and other healthcare and health policy professionals, to easily follow toward completing one's own literature review and synthesis. We attempt to include the many types of literature reviews that commonly provide information for healthcare professionals. While systematic reviews are imperative to clinical decision-making, we highlight other types of literature reviews that are essential to holistically incorporating multiple study types and diverse forms of information. We provide references to well-known as well as lesser-known resources that inform the literature review and synthesis process.

We provide a step-by-step overview of the process of conducting a literature review and synthesis. First, we have you identify the literature review and synthesis team members, while defining the topic area and establishing a specific review question. We then provide instructions for writing the review protocol. Next come the steps of conducting the review, including determining the eligibility criteria, search strategy, and databases, and then using that information to search the literature. Once that has been accomplished, the literature needs to be screened to determine if it meets inclusion criteria, critically appraised, and then, the data extracted. At the core of the process is synthesizing and creating new knowledge—which is no small task or accomplishment. Finally, we provide guidance on opportunities to disseminate your literature review. We also include references that detail the varied steps of the literature review process, allowing quick access to compare our recommendations against the processes of others, using multiple review types.

We hope that this book finds a place on your shelf, where it will be pulled out for a quick brush up of particular guidance on conducting each step of a literature review and synthesis. We also hope that the book becomes filled with your own notations, sticky notes, bookmarks, and bent corner pages that will further guide you as you are completing your own literature reviews and syntheses. We are all diversely motivated in our pursuits and commitments as healthcare professional students and learners, each in our own ways improving the health of the small and big worlds around us. The process of completing a literature review and synthesis can be foundational to improving our own knowledge, as well as enhancing understanding for those for whom it matters most. We wish you all the best in your individual and team pursuits to create and disseminate rigorous and meaningful literature reviews and syntheses to the global literature.

With gratitude,
Susan W. Buchholz and Kirsten A. Dickins

Acknowledgments

No book is ever written in isolation but rather with the consultation of pivotal experts. With that, we wish to thank those who provided vital knowledge that informed the content of this book, including Dr. Lou Fogg, Dr. Dola Pathak, Dr. George Kwabena Afari, Dr. Todd Ruppar, and Dr. Barbara Swanson. We also thank Jennifer Westrick and Talia DeGrazia for their assistance. We are grateful for your expertise and generosity that has helped to shape this book.

Acknowledgment

1 Introduction to Literature Review and Synthesis

Susan W. Buchholz and Kirsten A. Dickins

> *In an era shaped by appeals to emotion over science, and caprice over facts, the need for reliable evidence is greater now than ever before. Researchers across the globe are answering this call to action.*

CHAPTER OUTLINE

- Objectives
- Literature Synthesis Embedded within the Literature Review Process
- The Global Importance of Literature Review and Synthesis
- A Brief History of Literature Reviews
- Key Characteristics of Literature Reviews and Syntheses
- Terminology Related to Literature Review and Synthesis
- Overview of the Steps of the Literature Review and Synthesis Process
- Identifying the Purposes for Literature Review and Synthesis
- Bloom's Taxonomy and Literature Review and Synthesis
- Literature Review and Synthesis Resources
- Activities
- Summary Points
- References

This chapter introduces the literature synthesis process, as embedded within the overarching literature review process. The chapter begins by orienting you, the reviewer, to how literature synthesis is an essential component of the broader literature review process, critical to creating knowledge and advancing understanding among nurses and other healthcare professionals. A brief history of the evolution of the literature review is provided and key characteristics of literature reviews and syntheses are identified. The terminology is defined, and the steps of the overarching literature review process are outlined. The reasons for conducting a literature review and synthesis are then described. Thereafter, the stages of literature review and synthesis are summarized, as they relate to Bloom's Taxonomy of educational learning objectives. Lastly, global resources that are frequently utilized by literature reviewers are highlighted.

LEARNING OBJECTIVES

In this chapter, we introduce to you, the reviewer, the basics of literature synthesis, within the context of the literature review process. By the end of this chapter, you will be able to:

- Describe how literature synthesis is an essential part of the literature review process
- Identify the importance of literature synthesis
- Discuss the history and evolution of literature reviews
- Identify the key characteristics of literature reviews and syntheses
- Define terminology relevant to literature review and synthesis
- Differentiate the steps of the literature review and synthesis process
- Describe the distinct purposes for completing a literature review and synthesis
- Apply Bloom's Taxonomy to the literature review and synthesis process
- Review resources available for the literature review and synthesis process

LITERATURE SYNTHESIS EMBEDDED WITHIN THE LITERATURE REVIEW PROCESS

It is often the case that nurses and other healthcare professionals are not explicitly taught the necessary skills to systematically locate and synthesize pertinent information. If underprepared to perform these increasingly valuable skills, nurses and other healthcare professionals may become frustrated, or perhaps worse, miss the pertinent information altogether (Brettle & Gambling, 2003). It is the intention of the writers of this text that by the end of your reading, you—a member of the next generation of nurses and other healthcare professionals—will be prepared to excel at effectively locating necessary information and will be a confident professional who is able to systematically synthesize and generate new knowledge. The purpose of this book is to provide an overview and to educate you, the reviewer, on the steps of conducting a literature review and synthesis. To be able to understand how to complete a literature synthesis, the researcher must first have a foundational grasp of all steps of the literature review process, as they flow in a logical sequence. Therefore, this first chapter focuses primarily on literature synthesis, embedding it as one component or step within the overarching literature review process.

THE GLOBAL IMPORTANCE OF LITERATURE REVIEW AND SYNTHESIS

In an era shaped by appeals to emotion over science and caprice over facts, the need for reliable evidence is greater now than ever before. Researchers across the globe are answering this call to action. Each year, over 3 million scientific articles are published (Johnson et al., 2018). As the internet and online databases have made a vast amount of information available very quickly, it can be challenging for you as a reviewer to keep pace with the speed of publications and the knowledge therein (Derish & Annesley, 2011). With the rapidity and volume of scientific article publication, conflicting results can occur, owing to methodological shortcomings, authorial bias, and results produced by chance (Petticrew & Roberts, 2006). Publication proliferation can be an ongoing difficulty for those who are attempting to ascertain answers to specific questions or remain aware of the knowledge development on particular topics, given the vastness of scientific knowledge available (Bettany-Saltikov & McSherry, 2016; Eden et al., 2011). Conflicting results across publications can render it even more problematic for experts and non-experts alike to make sense of and know what is true, accurate, and representative of best science. This is, ideally, where literature review, and specifically, literature synthesis, enter the scene.

Consolidating and Resolving Conflict Across Findings

It is the literature review and synthesis process that can help you to collate and make sense of ever-growing and oft-conflicting findings that exist in the expanding "stacks" of virtual evidence. Isolated or single study findings are often insufficient for the development of a comprehensive and accurate picture (Khan et al., 2011). The literature review and synthesis process addresses these problems through the integration of findings across studies into one combined report, which is ideally measured and balanced in its consideration of multiple perspectives and findings. Not only does an effective literature review and synthesis present to the reviewer the state of the science through conveying a more comprehensive picture, it also contributes to resolving conflicts across the evidence (Whittemore, 2005). This synthesized source, eventually, may serve as a go-to source for clinicians and researchers alike to orient themselves. Through carrying out a successful literature review and synthesis process, you, the reviewer will compare, contrast, and combine the multiplying piles of evidence into understandable knowledge. Through this process, the reviewer will synthesize information to transform it into that which is most useable by nurses and other healthcare professionals, weighing conflicting findings with strengths and weaknesses. With the capacity to guide you to resolve conflicts in the evidence, literature reviews and syntheses have become an increasingly sought-after resource to inform understanding and decision-making for many nurses and other healthcare professionals.

Streamlining the Knowledge Acquisition Process

In many circles, rigorous literature reviews with syntheses are now recognized to be the most reliable source of knowledge emanating from research (Clarke & Chalmers, 2018). A testament to this belief is the 10,000 systematic reviews that are published annually worldwide (Clarke, 2018; Clarke & Chalmers, 2018), with literature reviews often being frequently cited. Searching the literature for relevant information can not only demand a considerable amount of time, but the process can be confusing and frustrating. You may continue to identify only irrelevant information, or in some circumstances, locate more information than is reasonably manageable (Brettle & Gambling, 2003). Literature review and synthesis holds multifold and far-reaching potential to streamline information to create the knowledge that helps to inform pertinent research, practice, and policy decisions.

Leveraging Literature Review and Synthesis to Aid Decision-Making

Those who are making clinical or health policy-related decisions generally benefit from relatively low barrier access to the highest quality evidence. Reading well-conducted literature reviews and syntheses can aid decision-makers in recognizing the quality of existing studies, as well as providing a high-quality summary of the extant literature (Clarke & Chalmers, 2018). When attempting to update yourself on the current state of an issue or topic outside of your immediate knowledge sphere, using summary or synthesized review documents is often not only advantageous but necessary (Derish & Annesley, 2011; Pautasso, 2013; Tricco et al., 2018). As we now know, published literature reviews have widely become recognized as an accessible representation of evidence from varied sources and professional fields, which can inform clinical practice and decisions related to a designated topic (Bolderston, 2008). As you read on throughout this text, it will become apparent that literature synthesis is a critical and core component of a literature review, and often the most challenging section to generate. The literature review and synthesis processes, from start to finish, will necessitate you coming to understand the state of the science, realizing the breadth and depth—or in some circumstances, the paucity of evidence on a particular topic—poising yourself to next summarize key literature on a specific topic. Advancing along, you will be prepared to systematically investigate why separate studies that explore the same question may report differing findings, evaluate existing theories, and perhaps even propose new theories. Your literature review and synthesis can and hopefully will serve as the foundation for guiding future research directions and recommending clinical and policy interventions (Petticrew & Roberts, 2006).

A BRIEF HISTORY OF LITERATURE REVIEWS

The Beginnings

The terms *literature review* and *literature synthesis* are increasingly heard in nursing and other healthcare professional circles—praised as a vital process to gain understanding and contribute toward improving the state of the science. As nursing and other healthcare professionals, you will undoubtedly be tasked with either preparing or reading literature reviews and syntheses throughout the course of your careers. While the past 20 years have been characterized by increasingly popular forms of literature review and synthesis in nursing (Aveyard & Bradbury-Jones, 2019), it is easy to forget that these "novel" forms of literature review date back centuries (Chalmers et al., 2002; Clarke & Chalmers, 2018; Schick-Makaroff et al., 2016). In fact, the intellectual tradition of review and synthesis date back as far as the times of Aristotle (Cooper & Hedges, 2009). One of the earliest documented literature review processes is recorded from 1753 in James Lind's review of publications addressing scurvy, marked by a severe vitamin C deficiency. It was in this literature review that Lind searched through the literature and "moved a great deal of rubbish" (as cited in Chalmers et al., 2002, p. 14; Clarke & Chalmers, 2018, p. 121)—or as we might label this activity today, conducted a critical appraisal, including only the literature that met a certain quality threshold.

20th Century

By the 20th century, literature review and synthesis–in the sense in which these terms are currently understood–began its emergence (Chalmers et al., 2002). In the 1970s and 1980s, scholars began to invest more attention into the ever-increasing need to improve the evidence synthesis process (Pericic & Tanveer, 2019). This period, from 1970 to 1989, has been referred to as the **foundation period** (Hong & Pluye, 2018). It was circa mid-foundation period, around the late 1970s, that review articles were noted to have high citation rates and review journals benefited by having higher impact factors (Chalmers et al., 2002), representing the budding recognition of the value of the review article within scholarly journals and circles. By the 1980s, the field of research synthesis in health disciplines was growing in popularity. At this point, standards for the critical evaluation of research reviews were disseminated—that is, the established process of identifying, assessing, and synthesizing information (Chalmers et al., 2002).

By the 1990s, textbooks and landmark reviews were being published, advancing the scientific quality of reviews in the social and health-related sciences (Chalmers et al., 2002); this point in time was the **evidence-based movement** (Schick-Makaroff et al., 2016). With the foundation of the Cochrane Collaboration in 1993—intended to propel those in healthcare to organize a critical summary of relevant randomized controlled trials (Cochrane Training, 2021)—an unprecedented movement toward the literature synthesis process was ignited. The last decade of the 20th century was characterized by literature reviews primarily classified into two approaches: (1) "Cochrane style" review, rigorous and systematic, often incorporating quantitative evidence, and (2) "narrative review," more methodologically accepting, summarizing bodies of often qualitative evidence (Aveyard & Bradbury-Jones, 2019). Narrative reviews were and often are utilized in the completion of doctoral dissertations (Aveyard & Bradbury-Jones, 2019). The decade spanning from 1990 to 2000 is referred to as the **institutionalization period** (Hong & Pluye, 2018). Toward the end of the institutionalization period, in the late 1990s and early 2000s, began the emergence of other forms of review, which we continue to note through the present day.

21st Century

We are currently in the climate of the **diversification period,** beginning formally in 2001 and extending through the present (Hong & Pluye, 2018). Some attribute the proliferation and variance in review types to a response to the earlier established division or dichotomy between the Cochrane-style review and narrative review. While part and parcel to the development and institutionalization of secondary research as an equally important form of research, these limited forms of review did not offer consideration of the various types of reviews that researchers desired, which included diverse primary study types. In the diversification period, new review types now offered alternative approaches to the Cochrane style, which allowed researchers to include varied primary study designs beyond the randomized controlled trial (Aveyard & Bradbury-Jones, 2019). Firmly into the diversification period of the 21st century, an even greater recognition of the importance of evidence, in conjunction with technological developments allowing ease in accessing online databases, has led to an uncharted proliferation in the publication of systematic and other types of reviews (Clarke & Chalmers, 2018). In addition, methods to combine primary studies progressed (Whittemore, 2005). While the systematic review is most closely associated with designing evidence-based practice initiatives, various types and studies emanating from diverse research methodologies, from quasi-experimental to qualitative studies, are also recognized and accepted as valuable to nursing and other health professional practices (Whittemore, 2005). At this current juncture, with this proliferation of research and knowledge, it is now more imperative than ever that literature reviews and syntheses be completed in accordance with the highest quality standards to inform healthcare practice and policy decision-making (Clarke & Chalmers, 2018). Moreover, reviewers must consistently relay quality criteria, toward the end of enhancing methodological rigor, and thereby confidence in conclusions and applicability of findings to practice (Whittemore, 2005).

KEY CHARACTERISTICS OF LITERATURE REVIEWS AND SYNTHESES

While there are many different types of literature reviews that require literature synthesis, such as systematic reviews, integrative reviews, rapid reviews, and so forth, literature reviews have differing characteristics. While there is not one particular framework that is accepted globally to identify characteristics of literature reviews, there are several expert classifications that guide the reviewer in understanding the fundamental aspects of a review. Due to a lack of overlap between different classification systems, it is useful to understand each classification system within its own context. Tables 1.1, 1.2, and 1.3 detail literature review classification systems (Cooper, 1985; Gough et al., 2012; Littell, 2018).

Although experts classify different aspects of engaging in the literature review and synthesis process, the similar contribution is the provision of foundational information used as organizational strategies for the following questions (Box 1.1).

In reviewing these questions, it is critical that the reviewer has a solid understanding of why the review is being conducted. With a firm understanding of why, or the rationale for conducting the literature review and synthesis, the groundwork is laid for

TABLE 1.1 CHARACTERISTICS OF LITERATURE REVIEWS (COOPER, 1985)

Focus	The review focus is the material in which the reviewer has a central interest.
Goal	The goals are what the reviewer hopes that the review will be able to accomplish.
Perspective	The perspective is the viewpoint that the reviewer uses in the discussion of the literature.
Coverage	Coverage is the extent to which the reviewer can locate and use relevant works.
Organization	Organization is how the review is arranged (e.g., historically, conceptually, methodologically).
Audience	The audience is the reviewer's intended readers.

TABLE 1.2 AGGREGATIVE AND CONFIGURATIVE REVIEW CONTINUA OF APPROACHES (GOUGH ET AL., 2012)

Philosophy	Idealist philosophical approach compared to realist philosophical approach.
Relation to theory	Generate theory, explore theory, test theory.
Approach to synthesis	Configuring results and/or aggregating results.
Methods	Using an iterative method or a priori method; using a theoretical search or an exhaustive search.
Quality assessment	Values the study contributions as compared to avoiding bias.
Products	Offers emerging concepts as compared to magnitude and precision.
Review uses	Used for enlightenment as compared to used instrumentally.

TABLE 1.3 COMPREHENSIVE SYSTEM FOR CLASSIFICATION OF RESEARCH REVIEWS (LITTELL, 2018)

Domain	The review topic is in one of the broad domains of conditions, interventions, or methodology.
Topics	The topic for the review is classified by the type of inferences being explored.
Goals	The goals reflect the review aims and the expectations that the reviewer is striving to accomplish.
Planning	Planning for the review is either a priori or taking an iterative approach.
Coverage	Coverage of studies to include can be either exhaustive, representative, purposive, or selective and incomplete.
Data types	Multiple sources of data can be part of a review, including quantitative, qualitative, individual participant data, or previous reviews.
Analysis and synthesis methods	The different types of analytical and synthesis methods can be used to configure and/or aggregate information.
Organization	The review can be organized historically, conceptually, or methodologically (Cooper, 1985).
Updating plans	Updates are planned at periodic time points or may be ongoing (Elliott et al., 2017).
Products/audiences	Dependent on the audience, the review may be a plain language summary, a brief report, or a full technical report.

BOX 1.1 QUESTIONS THAT PROVIDE ORGANIZATIONAL STRATEGIES FOR LITERATURE REVIEWS AND SYNTHESES

- Why am I conducting this review?
- What am I attempting to accomplish with this review?
- What will be included in the review?
- How will the review material be located?
- How will the review material be synthesized?
- How will the review material be organized?
- Who is the intended audience of the review?
- How will the review be disseminated?

---

what the reviewer decides to include, and the strategy used to complete a literature review and synthesis. Determination of the literature review and synthesis process, as well as the categorization or arrangement of materials follow next. One must note, however, that a literature review and synthesis holds little scientific meaning if not shared or disseminated in an appropriate venue with the people who can benefit most from seeing its findings.

TERMINOLOGY RELATED TO LITERATURE REVIEW AND SYNTHESIS

As the field of literature review and synthesis has grown, so have the options for language to describe the concepts central to these processes. Though the expanding breadth and depth of approaches may add richness to the process and outcomes, variance has come at the expense of uniformity (Schick-Makaroff et al., 2016). Proliferation without definition and categorization of terms has resulted in a lack of clarity about what characterizes each approach. While the term *literature synthesis* (as well as *evidence synthesis* and *research synthesis*) is often used interchangeably with the term *literature review,* these terms do not represent identical processes, but rather have both subtly and substantially different meanings (Cooper & Hedges, 2009). The struggle with the lack of global uniformity in the use of terminology relates to the lack of definitional consensus, even across academic domains. This consensus is further limited by the overlapping nature of the dimensions or categories across which literature reviews vary (Gough et al., 2012). This lack of consensus around identifying definitions of key terms used in the research literature is not a new problem and is linked to the jingle/jangle fallacy (Pedhazur & Schmelkin, 1991). The jingle fallacy represents the inaccurate belief that if two things have the same name, then they are the same thing even if the meanings of those things are different. The jangle fallacy represents the inaccurate belief that if two things have different names, even if they are identical in meaning, then they are inherently different.

It is important and arguably necessary to delineate how separate but related terms are characterized, what makes each term unique and worthy of its own definition, and what ties each term to the literature review and synthesis process altogether. There are many terms that are related to the literature review and synthesis processes, as well as different definitions that are provided for each construct. In this introductory chapter, we provide working definitions of key terms, including terms close in proximity to literature review and synthesis. Here, we have built upon the work of previous literature review and synthesis scholars to outline relevant term definitions.

Literature Synthesis

We have purposefully chosen to use the term *literature synthesis* as the distinct focus of this book. Although we discuss the *literature review* process, as we intend to cover the steps required to search, collect, review, and appraise the literature, we have highlighted the intended outcome of this work: the capacity to *synthesize* and generate new knowledge. Whether this new knowledge contributes meta-analytic scientific findings, meta-synthesis scientific findings, frameworks, directions for next steps, or other forms of knowledge, we believe that it is the *literature synthesis,* as part of the literature review process, that poises nurses and other healthcare and health policy professionals to create and offer valuable scientific contributions.

In this book, the term *literature synthesis* refers to the process of obtaining information from multiple sources, evaluating the ascertained information, and combining this information in unique ways to inform novel ways of understanding. It is an iterative process, necessitating the collection, review, and analysis of literature, with the goal of generating new concepts or theories, which may change and require revision over time. The synthesis process is not a simplistic one, but rather requires higher-order thinking: integration of decision-making, analytic, and evaluation skills, along with the capacity to generate new ideas informed by already established ideas (Shellenbarger, 2016). A literature synthesis compares data from primary literature, provides assessment of the quality of the studies, what and who were studied, and what the findings of the study were, examining potentially conflicting results. Building upon the synthesized review of the findings of the literature, the reviewer can examine strengths, limitations, implications, and gaps in the literature. A reviewer selects one of many approaches to synthesis, such as a quantitative or qualitative synthesis, depending upon the data type used (Schick-Makaroff et al., 2016). A thoughtfully completed literature synthesis can contribute to building new theories and frameworks, provide direction on how to implement a project or research study, as well as identify what topics or questions have not yet been fully examined and require more attention (Cooper & Hedges, 2009; Granello, 2001; Shellenbarger, 2016; Torraco, 2005). Figure 1.1 depicts the relationship of literature synthesis to other key literature review terms. A reviewer would find it challenging to complete a literature synthesis in isolation, as a literature synthesis is typically part of the larger literature review process. A reviewer may choose to complete a literature review, but may not include a literature synthesis. However, choosing to not include a

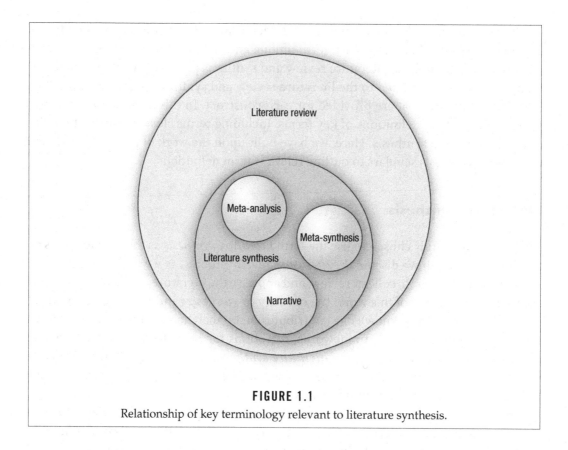

FIGURE 1.1

Relationship of key terminology relevant to literature synthesis.

literature synthesis would decrease the overall usability and meaningfulness of the literature review, as the synthesis is core to the contribution of the literature.

Evidence Synthesis

Evidence synthesis is a form of *literature synthesis,* which incorporates the processes of identifying, selecting, and combining results. *Evidence synthesis* is a method that examines data from relevant literature to answer a specific research question intended to be used to inform decision-making. Synthesized evidence is used to inform decision-making in healthcare practice and policy (Patient-Centered Outcomes Research Institute [PCORI], 2019). When a question arises, conducting an evidence synthesis allows for the careful examination of high-quality data sources to provide new or updated answers, as well as review recent data to highlight discordance or verify concordance with prior evidence synthesis reports. The steps of conducting an *evidence synthesis* are similar to the steps of *literature synthesis.*

Research Synthesis

A *research synthesis* is also broadly similar to a *literature synthesis,* as well as an *evidence synthesis,* referring to a process of locating, choosing, and integrating results. The primary focus and goal of *research synthesis* is to integrate empirical research for the purpose of creating generalizations, as well as setting the limits of these generalizations (Cooper & Hedges, 2009). A research synthesis involves a host of integrative activities, is attentive to relevant theories, critically analyzes included research, mediates conflicts in the research literature, and sets forth future research directions (Cooper & Hedges, 2009). The steps of conducting a *research synthesis* are similar to the steps of conducting a *literature synthesis*, and therefore also to the steps of an *evidence synthesis*.

Literature Review

In this text, the term *literature review* refers to a process whereby the reviewer examines, to varying degrees, the relevant literature on a chosen topic. The term *literature review* continues to be used broadly in academic, practice, and policy arenas, often as a generic term. In order to be classified as a *literature review*, two criteria must be met. A literature review generally must first use primary studies or database reports, and, second, offer descriptions, summaries, evaluations, clarifications, and integration of those sources (Cooper, 1985). There are some exceptions to this rule (e.g., umbrella reviews). When using the term *literature review*, the reviewer should ensure that a formalized examination of the existing scholarship in their area of inquiry has been completed. *Literature reviews* are one of the most important research methods, in the sense that a rigorously conducted *literature review* enables the researcher to determine the state of the literature in a given area of investigation (Galvan & Galvan, 2017). The term *literature review* is often used to describe what is done to provide background information for students' papers, including masters' theses and doctoral'dissertations and projects (Galvan & Galvan, 2017). The term *literature review* is also used by individuals who are not students, to explain the process undergone to examine a specific body of literature. The results of the *literature review* may inform a background section of the paper, a research study, a clinical decision, clinical guidelines, or a policy decision.

Systematic Review

A *systematic review* is a highly rigorous form of a *literature review* that aims to provide conclusions based on an exhaustive, formalized, and stepwise search of the literature. A *systematic review*, by definition, should be replicable. In a *systematic review*, literature is critically appraised to determine whether the quality of the literature is strong enough for inclusion in the analysis and synthesis of the findings. The *systematic review* process is used to control for or reduce bias when searching the literature, extracting data, and synthesizing the data (Chalmers et al., 2002). Dependent on the type of data sources that are included in a *systematic review*, as well as the type of findings available in the primary sources of data, a *systematic review* may or may not include a meta-analysis or meta-synthesis of the results. A *systematic review* can be a type of comparative effectiveness research when comparing alternative treatments, which provides the benefits of including a large number of participants; the *systematic review* includes results at the population level as well as the subgroup level, positive and negative outcomes, and can reflect clinical settings (Eden et al., 2011).

Meta-Analysis

A *meta-analysis* is not a *systematic review* but is often a core part of a *systematic review* that is includes quantitative studies (Little et al., 2008). A *meta-analysis* is a statistical approach to analyzing quantitative results of one or more variables from two or more primary data sources. Different quantitative procedures are used in the *meta-analysis* process to statistically combine individual study results, using for example, forest plots (Cooper & Hedges, 2009; Lewis & Clarke, 2001). A *meta-analysis* is part of the synthesis process, in that this statistical procedure examines quantitative results from more than one source of data to establish a new set of aggregated results.

Meta-Synthesis

A *meta-synthesis* is not a *systematic review* but can be a core part of a *systematic review* that is comprised of qualitative studies. Broadly, a *meta-synthesis* is the process of synthesizing qualitative studies. It is worth noting that there are several terms used to describe the process of synthesizing qualitative studies, such as *qualitative evidence synthesis* (Noyes et al., 2019). There are different methodological processes used in the synthesis of qualitative literature, for example, meta-aggregation, meta-ethnography, or thematic synthesis.

Narrative

The *narrative* component of a *literature synthesis* is where results of the synthesis are conveyed in text or paragraph format. The *narrative* component of the review is often accompanied by a table in which the reviewer expands on their interpretation of the results. If there is no table and no statistical or qualitative methodological analysis, then a *literature review* may be written only in text or paragraph format, in which the reviewer describes the individual studies as well as the synthesized results of the studies. In the *narrative* component of a literature review, results of data extraction are compared and contrasted and then synthesized to present an aggregated representation of what the literature or data sources mean as a whole (Petticrew & Roberts, 2006).

Review

The term *review*, used alone without any specific descriptor, can also be noted in the literature. However, when the term *review* is used by itself, it can be difficult to discern exactly what the reviewer did, or how the *review* was completed. A *review* conveys only that some type of exploration of the literature was completed, without suggestion or guarantee that the *review* was systematized, formalized, or exhaustive. Nor does the term *review* indicate the rationale, scope, or interpretation for why the review was undertaken. Therefore, the term *review* is dependent on the context in which it is used. If a reviewer states that they have completed a *review*, for example, a clinical review, or a review of the literature within a scholarly paper, the reviewer may have grossly examined the literature to create a baseline understanding and provide background information on a particular topic or question. If a *clinical review* has been completed, then the reviewer may have selected certain clinical articles to inform their work. Therefore, when a reader sees the word *review* used alone, the task falls to the reader to assess how and what level of rigor was applied to the *review*.

Annotated Bibliography

An *annotated bibliography* is comprised of a list of citations from various sources, including articles, books, and other data sources, followed by a brief descriptive overview of each source, generally about one paragraph in length. When a reviewer prepares an *annotated bibliography*, they are summarizing and reporting on each separate data source. Each data source is evaluated for specific purposes, which is determined by the reviewer and their review question and purpose. Dependent on the purpose of the *annotated bibliography*, the summary will descriptively overview each data source, comment on its contribution to the area of focus, and provide a brief evaluation. Unlike a *literature synthesis*, in an *annotated bibliography*, there is no synthesis of the data sources, but rather a separate reporting of each source (Bolderston, 2008).

Primary Research in Relation to Literature Review and Synthesis

The literature review and synthesis process bring together primary research for the purpose of creating new knowledge. Primary research is the process of conducting an original research study to answer a specific question. The literature review process is associated with the review and synthesis of quantitative and/or qualitative primary research (e.g., systematic reviews, integrative reviews). With the literature review process, the reviewer is not conducting a primary study but rather generating knowledge through the review and synthesis of published literature, as well as unpublished literature that is relevant to the review.

OVERVIEW OF THE STEPS OF THE LITERATURE REVIEW AND SYNTHESIS PROCESS

Regardless of the type of literature review and synthesis being conducted, the core steps for conducting the review and synthesizing the literature share critical features, though recommendations from experts include different numbers of and emphases within the

---

BOX 1.2   THE PROCESS OF CONDUCTING A LITERATURE REVIEW LEADING TO A LITERATURE SYNTHESIS

- Identify literature review and synthesis team members
- Define the topic area, establish a specific review question
- Write the review protocol
- Determine the eligibility criteria, search strategy, and databases
- Search the literature
- Screen the literature
- Critically appraise the literature
- Extract the data
- Synthesize and create new knowledge
- Disseminate your literature review and synthesis

---

required steps (Aromataris & Munn, 2017; Conn & Coon Sells, 2014; Eden et al., 2011; Higgins & Thomas, 2021; Pautasso, 2013). In this text we overview the steps (Box 1.2) offered by literature review experts, outlining the process to occur when conducting a careful literature review and synthesis of the data. While each of the steps in the process is pertinent, there is some flexibility in the depth at which these steps might be undertaken by each reviewer. In other words, you need to determine how you are going to apply these steps based on the purpose and question of your literature review and synthesis. With that in mind, whatever permutation of steps that you select, it is essential for you to follow a systematized, protocol-driven process in order to guarantee that the review and synthesis process is organized and rigorous and that the results are trustworthy and based on standardized guidelines.

Following the literature review and synthesis process steps sequentially is recommended in order to make certain that you have conducted a comprehensive review that does not exclude relevant data or include inappropriate data. Each of the steps in the literature review process are examined in further depth in upcoming chapters. The purpose of this initial overview is to serve as a high-level orientation to the major steps involved in conducting a systematized, organized literature review and synthesis.

Identify Literature Review and Synthesis Team Members

One may begin by carefully considering and determining who is an optimal member of the literature review and synthesis team ("review team"; Aromataris & Munn, 2017). Each review team member should have the capacity to contribute unique perspectives, recognizing the diversity of team member backgrounds as distinct strengths. Typically, at least two people—or more, if additional expertise is needed—will participate in all steps of the literature review and synthesis process. To avoid confusion or losing time in determining who is primarily responsible for the review process, one person should be designated as the review team leader. If a review is being completed quickly to inform a specific topic such as in the setting of a rapid review, it may possibly be undertaken by only one person, though we strongly encourage you to consider and acknowledge in advance the limitations of completing a one-person review. While a review completed by one person might be useful in providing background information on a topic, informing methodological considerations, or supporting the discussion section of a manuscript, the literature review likely would not be sufficiently rigorous to constitute a formal literature review and synthesis suitable for publication. There may be times when the researcher puts together the team after sthey have fully determined what question the reviewer is aiming to answer. For example, this may occur when a graduate student conducts several preliminary searches of the literature to identify the gaps in the literature, or to assess if literature reviews have already been published on the topic/question of interest. If the graduate student finds that their question has recently been answered in an already published literature review, then the graduate student may shift, expand, or narrow the focus of the original question, which may necessitate reformation of the review team.

Define the Topic Area, Establish a Specific Review Question

How you begin your approach to the literature review and synthesis process will be unique to you and your set of interests and expertise. However, first and foremost, you will need to identify a topic area, which will inform the development of the purpose and question of your literature review and synthesis. Often the purpose is related to a question that you have been contemplating or a topic that you have wanted to better understand. The topic may be informed by your area of clinical, research, or policy expertise, or possibly a side project that has been puzzling you or calling for your attention. After you decide on your topic or area of interest, you will determine the purpose of the review, then craft a clear and specific review question. The review purpose and question will be core to the entirety of the literature review and synthesis, the guidepost that you will continue to revisit to keep you oriented. The review purpose, informed by your topic or area of interest, will drive the formulation and framing of the review question. The population, intervention, control, and outcomes (PICO) format for quantitative research and the PICO format for qualitative research, are popular and respected methods used to frame literature review questions (Lockwood et al., 2020; Thomas et al., 2019). The type of literature review and synthesis that you ultimately undertake will stem from the nature of the review question.

Write the Review Protocol

The protocol for the literature review provides a roadmap for you and your review team that will be continually revisited when conducting the literature review and synthesis. This is the document that serves as the formal "guide to the review" for every review team member, ranging anywhere in skill and experience from novice to expert. A protocol written on conducting a formal literature review is typically extensive, including strategies for searching the literature, selecting data sources, critically appraising data sources, and outlining an analytic plan. The protocol is always written using a systematic format, regardless of the reason for conducting a literature review and synthesis. For certain organizations, protocols are required and peer-reviewed prior to beginning the literature review and synthesis process (Aromataris & Munn, 2017; Lasserson et al., 2019). If you intend to publish your literature review and synthesis, the protocol may require formal registration (e.g., PROSPERO), if not already published with an organization that guides systematic reviews (PROSPERO, 2019).

Determine the Eligibility Criteria, Search Strategy, and Databases

Next, you will establish eligibility criteria to begin to provide the parameters or determine what you might include versus exclude in your search. Determining which inclusion and exclusion criteria (termed: eligibility criteria) will be used when screening retrieved texts will create limitations so that a literature review is focused and manageable. Determining the keywords that will be used in your search strategy results from a careful process of knowing and selecting most commonly used terminology, dependent on your discipline, topic, review purpose and question, and selected databases. Utilizing Medical Subject Heading (MeSH) terms and trees—often under the guidance of a healthcare librarian—can help you to systematically determine the terms that will yield the most comprehensive and accurate results, including those that are not formal MeSH terms. Deciding where (databases) and how (strategy) you will search the literature, or creating a "search strategy" to be employed in select databases, is necessary to comprehensively locate the most fitting literature available to address a review purpose and question (Eden et al., 2011; Littell et al., 2008). Toward this end, the reviewer needs to systematically determine which words and phrases will be used to search the literature, otherwise known as the development of a formal "search strategy." While it is helpful to be affiliated with an academic institution or another setting in which expert support for search strategy development and execution is available, if this is not possible, you may benefit from working closely with other researchers with experience in creating and executing a search strategy. In order to execute the search strategy, you will also select the databases that will be accessed and used. To select databases, you will first need to have a solid understanding of which databases are relevant to your review purpose and question. While popular databases such as PubMed and Google Scholar exist in the public domain, there are hundreds of other databases available primarily for professional research use.

Search the Literature

After determining the eligibility criteria, creating the search strategy, and selecting the databases, you are now ready to formally execute the search. This is the point at which the search strategy is applied to and exercised within the identified databases (Eden et al., 2011;

Littell et al., 2008). If you have access to collaborate with a healthcare librarian or other literature review expert, this individual will most optimally guide you through this phase. Once the search is executed, the ease with which you will be able to retrieve the literature is in part related to resources to which you have access, including peer-reviewed literature as well as grey literature. Obtaining all of the identified sources of data for an initial search can be challenging. We recommend that you have a data access plan in place to ensure that you will be able to retrieve full texts of any potentially eligible literature. You also need to determine how you will store the retrieved literature. For example, cataloging electronic articles using reference management software is a common strategy in more recent literature reviews, while some reviewers prefer to print paper copies of retrieved articles. Whichever approach you choose to retrieve and store the literature, also consider ease of access to this literature by all members of the review team.

Screen the Literature

Once the search is executed and the literature is retrieved, you will then assess eligibility of the literature using several phases of screening (Lefebvre et al., 2019). Depending on your resources, your review team may or may not use an online literature review platform, such as Covidence, to organize and sequence the multi-step literature screening process. While some review teams may use a hand screening method with printed literature, online literature review platforms are a contemporary, user-friendly option that are easily and quickly accessed by users working in different locations. During the multi-step screening phase, establishing eligibility (inclusion/exclusion) criteria will guide your review team's determinations. In a rigorous literature review, a dual-blinded screening will occur, initially of the titles then abstracts, or more likely, of titles and abstracts together. Once it is determined whether titles and abstracts meet or do not meet eligibility criteria, you will then move to screening full texts of the remaining eligible articles. In the full-text screening phase, each remaining article is considered in its entirety, independently by each of the two reviewers. At the end of each step of the screening phase, the two reviewers should come together to discuss their decisions and resolve any differences of opinion regarding an eligibility determination. A third party may be required to help adjudicate eligibility determination discrepancies. For reviews that are completed to inform the background of a manuscript which are not part of a formal literature review, a single reviewer may choose to screen the literature themselves and not require this final step of adjudication.

Critically Appraise the Literature

Reviewers must follow a rigorous process for carefully reading and critically appraising the literature that has been deemed eligible for inclusion in the review (Critical Appraisal Skills Programme, 2018). Prior to starting the search of the literature, the reviewer should determine what is important regarding quality of the article, and which criteria will be used to determine if the article meets or does not meet the predetermined quality threshold. After the title, abstract, and full-text screening steps are completed and you have determined which literature meet the eligibility criteria, you must then appraise the literature to assess quality. There are different critical appraisal tools available to guide the determination of whether an article should be formally included or discarded based on evidence quality. Fortunately, the several critical appraisal tools available allow you to select one that fits well with the purpose of the literature review and synthesis. If you are working with a specific review organization, then it will likely be suggested for you to use that organization's recommended critical appraisal tool. When literature is less formally searched and collected to answer a question, you will still need to methodically appraise the literature to determine whether it is indeed accurate and reliable. Whichever tool you choose to assess the quality of the included literature, you will need to document and explicitly describe the appraisal process in your literature review and synthesis write-up.

Extract the Data

After you have determined which literature meets eligibility criteria and quality appraisal thresholds, you will undergo the stepwise, detailed process of data extraction. Various data extraction tools exist, suited to different types of research study designs, as well as other types of literature such as expert opinion articles, that you will be including as the data sources in your literature review and synthesis (Garrard, 2017; Lockwood et al., 2020; McArthur et al., 2020; Tufanaru et al., 2020). If you are working with a specific organization, then you will likely use the data extraction tools specific to that organization. However, if you are working independently, you may then choose to use an established tool or decide to create your own data extraction sheet or table. Traditionally, data extraction has been completed using author-developed tools such as typing the information into a word processing document on a computer. However, there is now sophisticated and user-friendly software designed specifically for the data extraction phase of a literature review. Whether you are using an established data extraction tool or an author-developed data extraction tool, it is helpful to choose a tool or multiple tools that allow you to extract the data that will answer in a way most fitting to your distinct review purpose and question.

Synthesize and Create New Knowledge

Finally, you are ready to synthesize the literature. You can begin by carefully revisiting findings that you have extracted into your data sheets from the included literature and data sources (Cooper, 2017; Littell et al., 2008; McKenzie et al., 2019). While each of the steps of the literature review and synthesis process will demand attention to detail, the synthesis step is generally the step that researchers find most intellectually challenging. You may first report independent main article results, often in a tabular format, which will then be followed by a literature synthesis in narrative format. This is also the point at which you may complete a meta-analysis or meta-synthesis, if applicable to your review purpose, question, and type of data available. The literature synthesis process tasks reviewers with comparing and contrasting what they have found, looking for similarities and differences, as well as missing data or gaps in the included literature. While up until this point you have been making determinations about what literature and data sources should be included in the literature review and synthesis, you will now have to see beyond each individual source to envision what all of the findings mean in aggregate, creating a whole picture. This requires curiosity, time, refined critical thinking capacity, and the ability to comprehend what a single piece of literature means in relation to its companion literature.

Disseminate Your Literature Review and Synthesis

The final step is an essential one, that of dissemination (Bettany-Saltikov & McSherry, 2016; Petticrew & Roberts, 2006). When preparing for dissemination, you need to allow for sufficient time to craft an explanatory title, write an inclusive and easily understood abstract, and choose keywords that will allow others to find your work (which may or may not overlap with the terms and phrases used in your search strategy). You will also need to carefully explore where and how you want to disseminate your work. If you do not report and provide implications on your literature review findings, then your contribution will be lost to the scientific and lay community. Where and how you as the reviewer determine to report your literature review findings will in part limit or expand the possibilities for other people to locate, learn from, and ultimately use your literature review to inform their own work and scientific contributions. Providing thoughtful and succinct implications of the findings can be very useful for the readers in helping them to determine their own future directions.

IDENTIFYING THE PURPOSES FOR LITERATURE REVIEW AND SYNTHESIS

Researchers conduct literature syntheses for a variety of reasons, as depicted in Box 1.3.

The literature synthesis process is intended to provide a trustworthy answer to a specific question (Booth et al., 2016). Using a rigorous scientific process, information can be gathered from around the globe about a specific topic, in order to determine what is known or not known about a subject (Bolderston, 2008; Fink, 2020). The synthesis of this literature can provide the background and rationale for conducting new research (Brettle & Gambling, 2003). A literature synthesis is a vital component of manuscripts, theses, and dissertations that are conducted as partial fulfillment of specific academic degrees (Bolderston, 2008; Fink, 2020), and can be an integral element of a course of study for nurses (Timmins & McCabe, 2005) and other healthcare and health policy professionals. Immersing oneself in the generation of a literature synthesis increases awareness of existing research, its implications, and potential future

---

BOX 1.3   REASONS FOR CONDUCTING A LITERATURE REVIEW AND SYNTHESIS

- Offers trustworthy answers to a specific question
- Provides a reference for readers interested in broadening and deepening their knowledge of specific critical issues
- Evaluates the strengths, weaknesses, and overall quality of available evidence
- Identifies areas of controversy and debate
- Reveals the level of consistency and discordance of findings across multiple studies
- Brings readers up-to-date with a distillation of the literature
- Provides statistical data to inform decision-making
- Identifies and calls attention to gaps in knowledge that require further investigation
- Attempts to systematically address conscious and unconscious bias in research

---

directions (e.g., becoming familiar with research studies, terminology, methodology; Timmins & McCabe, 2005). Literature synthesis is also a helpful process and contribution when writing funding proposals for research or program planning, development, or evaluation (Fink, 2020).

A literature synthesis provides an updated reference for readers who are interested in broadening their knowledge of critical issues, also serving as a tool for intellectual enrichment and enhancement of research standards (Liumbruno et al., 2013). Literature syntheses often include a list, typically in a tabular format of the studies and other data sources that comprised the materials used in the data synthesis. Literature from around the globe can be located in one central place that the reviewer can quickly view and determine who are the researchers; what, with whom, where, and how was it studied; and what was found out as a result of the study.

While it is important to know what literature is available on a topic, it is equally important to uncover the strength and quality of available evidence (Booth et al., 2016). The critical appraisal process assesses the quality of the study and review or narrative writings from which the literature synthesis is created. Formal and psychometrically tested tools exist to aid the reviewer in the process of critically appraising the literature (Critical Appraisal Skills Programme, 2018; Joanna Briggs Institute, 2021). After a critical appraisal of each data source is completed, the reviewer determines if the quality is sufficient in order to move the data source on to the next step of extracting information to be used in the review. Vetted data sources that are used for the synthesis provide the reviewer with a high quality of literature to inform decision-making at the healthcare practice and policy levels.

Additionally, through literature synthesis, a reviewer can identify areas of controversy and debate (Bolderston, 2008). Results from a literature synthesis may surprise the professional and lay communities and can bring about a shift in common practices. Literature syntheses may show conflicting findings on similar topics, causing the review community to closely analyze how the literature synthesis was executed. Reading different types of literature reviews, including systematic reviews that have included a literature synthesis, can serve as the basis for evidence-based practice (Brettle & Gambling, 2003; Fink, 2020). Organizations such as the Campbell Collaboration (2021) provide systematic reviews in areas that have high potential for debate, including crime and justice, international development, social welfare, as well as other areas with a broad societal reach regarding decision-making. Dependent on the societal context and the findings, the potential for identifying controversy can exist in any arena in which literature synthesis occurs.

Literature synthesis reveals the level of consistency of findings across multiple studies (Booth et al., 2016). For narrative data, the researcher can compare and contrast specific findings to assess for similarities and differences (Moola et al., 2017). Tabular data synthesis also provides a method for reviews to assess for consistency of findings in different studies (Moola et al., 2017). When appropriate, the researcher can compare data at a very high level of detail to assess whether findings are consistent across studies. For the meta-analysis component of the literature synthesis, the researcher is advised to use homogeneous data conveying comparable outcomes. If the researcher uses heterogeneous data in a meta-analysis, then the researcher needs to provide a compelling explanation as to the inclusion of these data (Tufanaru et al., 2020) and how dissimilar outcomes were aggregated in comparable ways.

Because of the summary format, a literature synthesis can quickly bring reviewers up-to-date with current literature. Given the potential for a high volume of evidence on a given topic, literature syntheses distill the evidence to help students and professionals in a field to keep pace with a quickly growing knowledge base (Bettany-Saltikov & McSherry, 2016). This understanding can then be leveraged as justification for further research and action (Cronin et al., 2008). Given the vast amount of literature available globally in quickly accessed search engines, it can be challenging for professional and lay readers to have a well-rounded sense of the literature in more than a few topic areas. Literature reviews and syntheses allow for readers of all levels to quickly identify the state-of-the literature. For example, in the biomedical database search engine PubMed, there are over 32 million citations available (National Library of Medicine, 2021). PubMed allows readers to quickly locate different types of literature reviews that can be filtered by date.

When statistical results are presented as a component of literature synthesis, the results can provide for researchers, clinicians, and policymakers, an awareness of the statistical confidence needed to determine how to interpret and select compelling results for decision-making (Booth et al., 2016). Equally important is for the researcher, clinician, and policymaker to hone the skill of presenting statistical results in a manner interpretable by the lay public. Lay summaries are useful to include as part of scientific writings, so that the public has the ability to quickly comprehend an overview of the findings and make decisions informed by the review findings (Barnes & Patrick, 2019).

Methodically generating a literature synthesis is one safeguard to attempt to systematically subvert the natural tendency to be swayed by conscious and unconscious biases (e.g., pet theories, appeal to funders, perceived need to produce positive findings; Petticrew & Roberts, 2006). A high level of rigor should be applied to all litera-ture review processes, including the creation of the synthesis. The literature synthesis should include studies that accepted the null hypothesis (Mlinaric et al., 2017). There-fore, searching multiple data sources, including the grey literature, allows the reviewer to capture a wider breadth of the published and unpublished data (Mahood et al., 2014).

Important for future research, interpretation of the literature synthesis allows for the identification of gaps in knowledge that require further investigation (Booth et al., 2016). There can be a justification for new studies needed to fill in the gaps (Fink, 2020). Identification and formulation of future research questions can set the scene for a pri-mary research study (Bolderston, 2008). Recommendations provided as a result of the literature synthesis can give ideas on how to proceed with research (Brettle & Gam-bling, 2003). Literature syntheses acknowledge previously published work, while demon-strating that new research that is being undertaken is adding to the body of literature (Bolderston, 2008).

BLOOM'S TAXONOMY AND LITERATURE REVIEW AND SYNTHESIS

The skills that are necessary for you to create a strong literature review and synthesis (e.g., decision-making, analysis, evaluation, and development of new material) demonstrate significant overlap with the skills utilized in everyday nursing practice (Shellenbarger, 2016). However, the skills of synthesis, specifically, the creation of new material, is a skill that is often not explicitly taught. Educators may make assumptions regarding a stu-dent's ability to transfer the critical thinking skills of clinical practice into the critical thinking and technical writing skills required in the completion of a literature review and synthesis. Here we use the framework of Bloom's Taxonomy, emphasizing only the cognitive domain, to aid in explaining the learning objectives and trajectory as nursing and other health professional students build the knowledge and skill base required to prepare strong literature reviews and syntheses. Categories are based on the revised edition of Bloom's Taxonomy (2001) and are influenced by the thoughts and writings of Darcy Haag Granello (2001) and Matthew Iwuchukwu (2016).

Knowledge

Also known as "remembering," this first step in the learning process requires the acqui-sition of basic facts relevant to a particular topic. During the knowledge phase, while a student may not yet be capable of seeing or understanding the entire meaning of the knowledge that they are acquiring, the student is becoming able to recognize and recall important concepts. Throughout the knowledge acquisition phase, the learner is begin-ning to accumulate and organize information on a given topic. They search online data-bases, pull relevant online or in-print brooks, and review other relevant sources such as the grey literature, conference materials, popular media outlets, or related theses/

dissertations. Information may also come through conversation with advisors, mentors, or other key experts in their field of study.

Comprehension

Otherwise referred to as "understanding," the learner is becoming able to organize, interpret, and compare important ideas in the comprehension phase. The learner is now moving toward being able to independently offer descriptions of and clearly state the main ideas relevant to their topic. Comprehension is derived from immersion of oneself into the knowledge acquisition phase, equipping oneself with awareness and the ability to recognize empirical data and a wide range of perspectives on a given topic. During the comprehension phase, the learner draws upon the knowledge gained during the immediately prior phase to draw parallels, compare and contrast, and understand key ideas across the literature with a greater understanding of a deeper meaning of key constructs and ideas.

Application

In the application phase, the learner is now prepared to leverage newly ascertained knowledge and comprehension to apply facts, concepts, and ideas across novel situations to unique problems. The learner is able to form connections between new knowledge and comprehension, recognizing relations, and extrapolate skillfully to integrate awareness and understanding of ideas into new contexts. In the application phase, the learner is beginning to formulate an approach to undertaking their own literature review and synthesis, and to formulate a precise review purpose and question and inform a background section.

Analysis

The analysis phase involves awareness of how to cogently organize and examine all layers of information, separately and in aggregate. As part of the analysis, learners should be able to perform a critical evaluation (also known as a critical analysis) of the extant literature, identifying and succinctly conveying strengths and weaknesses. During the analysis phase, the learner should also become able to recognize the interrelations between different parts of information, formulate hypotheses regarding a topic, and integrate evidence to support these hypotheses.

Synthesis

In the synthesis phase, the learner has accumulated baseline knowledge that has informed their comprehension of a topic. They are now able to apply this comprehension in and across settings and analyze integral information. Throughout the synthesize phase, the learner becomes able to leverage the aforementioned steps to inform novel notions. The synthesis phase is also one of creation. During this phase, the learner begins by pulling together and integrating both similar and diverse ideas; from bringing together like and different ideas, the learner positions themselves to generate and offer a new idea. Whether this is calling attention to a discrepancy or a gap in the literature or pulling together a story not yet told by the aggregate data, the learner becomes capable of and responsible to create something fresh that has not yet been noted in the existing literature.

Evaluation

In the evaluation phase, the learner has officially engaged in exceptional self-transformation activities. They are transitioning from novice to becoming a topic or field expert. They move from building an arsenal of basic facts and concepts to positioning oneself to contribute innovative and important ideas to the scientific literature. Now, having gained knowledge, developed comprehension, began the process of applying this comprehension across settings, grew and refined analytic abilities, and created a meaningful synthesis, the learner is prepared to offer and substantiate their viewpoints, which are the results of their synthesis. With a conscientious awareness and critical eye toward both the new and dated scientific literature, the learner can thoughtfully formulate and share well-informed judgments or evaluations of the literature both now and moving forward. They can tactfully bring attention to the strengths and weaknesses of the science while empowering themselves to make the recommended changes.

It is our hope that as you, the reviewer, move through the different cognitive phases of Bloom's Taxonomy, while choosing to remain invested in your field of study, whether it be nursing or another healthcare or health policy profession. If you are able to do that, you will be able to more comprehensively remain abreast of relevant scientific advances. It is also our hope that you choose to continue to immerse yourself in this process on novel topics throughout your successful career.

LITERATURE REVIEW AND SYNTHESIS RESOURCES

There are a multitude of resources available globally at all levels that can be quickly accessed by reviewers via the internet. Some of these available resources require membership or affiliation with a professional organization or institution. Fortunately, even these organizations typically provide part of their resources freely to professionals and the lay public. Box 1.4 displays a relevant but non-exhaustive list of organizations and associated websites that provide different types of resources for conducting and serve as repositories for literature reviews and syntheses. In this introductory chapter, only a very brief description is given of these various centers, networks, and organizations. At each of these websites, there are myriad state-of-the-science resources available.

BOX 1.4   RESOURCES FOR CONDUCTING LITERATURE REVIEW AND SYNTHESIS*

- Africa Evidence Network
  - www.aen-website.azurewebsites.net
  - Pan-African network that contributes to ending poverty and inequity in Africa by increasing the use of evidence in decision-making.
- Centre for Evidence-Based Medicine Resources
  - www.cebm.net
  - United Kingdom Centre that supports the development, promotion, and dissemination of healthcare evidence.
- Centre for Reviews and Dissemination
  - www.york.ac.uk/crd
  - United Kingdom Centre that advances the use of research evidence for improving population health.
- Centres for Systematic Reviews of Health Policy and Systems Research in Low- and Middle-Income Countries
  - www.who.int/alliance-hpsr/projects/unicatolica_srccrosscutting/en
  - Chile-based organization supports Centres for systematic reviews of health policy and systems research in low-and middle-income countries.
- Cochrane Collaboration
  - www.cochrane.org
  - United Kingdom-based organization that produces systematic reviews and other synthesized research evidence.
- Evidence-Based Nursing
  - www.ebn.bmj.com
  - United Kingdom-based organization that searches international healthcare journals to locate valid and relevant research for best nursing practice.
- Finding What Works in Health Care
  - www.nap.edu/catalog/13059/finding-what-works-in-health-care-standards -for-systematic-reviews
  - United States Institute of Medicine reference provides healthcare decision-makers with standards for systematic reviews.
- Health Evidence Network
  - www.euro.who.int/en/data-and-evidence/evidence-informed-policy-making/ health-evidence-network-hen
  - World Health Organization and European network providing evidence for decision-making in healthcare.
- Joanna Briggs Institute
  - www.jbi.global

(continued)

> **BOX 1.4   RESOURCES FOR CONDUCTING LITERATURE REVIEW AND SYNTHESIS** (*continued*)
>
>   - Australia-based organization promotes and supports the use of best available evidence for healthcare decision-making at the point of care.
> - The Campbell Collaboration
>   - www.campbellcollaboration.org
>   - Norwegian-based network that provides policy-relevant evidence syntheses, plain language summaries, and policy briefs in the social sectors.
> - The Evidence for Policy and Practice Information and Coordinating Centre (EPPI-Centre)
>   - www.eppi.ioe.ac.uk/cms
>   - United Kingdom Centre that informs policy and professional practice by systematic review and research evidence use work.
>
> *URLs were live at the time of publication; however, URLs may change over time.

ACTIVITIES
Activity I

You are interested in reviewing literature reviews focused on the effects of dog ownership on cardiovascular disease. Please choose two systematic reviews to provide a beginning overview of the available literature reviews on the topic.

- Kramer, C. K., Mehmood, S., & Suen, R. C. (2019). Dog ownership and survival: A systematic review and meta-analysis. *Circulation: Cardiovascular Quality and Outcomes, 12*(10):e005554. doi: https://doi.org/10.1161/CIRCOUTCOMES.119.005554. Available at: www.ahajournals.org/doi/pdf/10.1161/CIRCOUTCOMES.119.005554

- Yeh, T. L., Lei, W. T., Liu, S. J., & Chien, K. L. (2019). A modest protective association between pet ownership and cardiovascular diseases: A systematic review and meta-analysis. *PLoS One, 14*(5):e0216231. doi: https://doi.org/10.1371/journal.pone.0216231. Available at: www.ncbi.nlm.nih.gov/pmc/articles/PMC6499429/pdf/pone.0216231.pdf

You note that the first review written by Kramer et al. (2019) studies dog ownership and cardiovascular survival. In their conclusion, they write that "Dog ownership is associated with lower risk of death over the long term, which is possibly driven by a reduction in cardiovascular mortality" (p. 1). The second review is by Yeh et al. (2019) and studies pets in general, including dogs, and cardiovascular disease. In their conclusion they write that "Pet ownership is not associated with adjusted all-cause or cardiovascular (CV) mortality, or risk of cardiovascular disease (CVD), myocardial infarction (MI), or stroke, but it is associated with a lower adjusted CV mortality in the general population and a lower CVD risk in patients with established CVD" (p. 1).

You read the reviews on dog and pet ownership in relationship to cardiovascular risk and disease in their entirety. Afterward, please answer the following questions.

1. What is the reason that the authors completed a literature review on this topic?
2. What are the literature review and synthesis steps that the reviewers followed?
3. What constitutes the literature synthesis components of these reviews?
4. Do you think the findings of these literature reviews are equivalent? Please explain your answer.
5. How could the findings of these literature reviews be used to inform decisions made by nurses and other healthcare and health policy professionals?

Activity II

As a nurse or other healthcare or health policy professional, please identify an area that you want to learn more about.

1. Write 3 to 5 sentences about what you already know and do not know about your selected topic area.
2. Identify why you want to study that area and write a potential review question.
3. Think into the future about how the literature review and synthesis that you contribute to that topic area could be used by other people. In what ways? What would the literature review and synthesis need to entail?

SUMMARY POINTS

We recognize the level of expertise already available on literature review and synthesis processes is extensive. We hope to draw upon this expertise throughout the remainder of this text, to bring together diverse and rich perspectives to make existing guidance more easily comprehensive and encourage your success in conducting impactful literature reviews and syntheses. With this, we are confident that you will use the literature review and synthesis process as an established and recognized form of knowledge generation to contribute to the advancement of nursing and healthcare and health policy professions science, and ultimately, to the improved health of humanity.

- Literature synthesis is a crucial component of the literature review process. To understand literature synthesis, a reviewer needs to have a working knowledge of the literature review process.
- Given the volume of literature that is published annually, it is becoming increasingly difficult for one researcher to read and comprehend more than a very narrow aspect of a given topic. Therefore, rigorously completed literature reviews and syntheses provide important and useful information for nurses and other healthcare and health policy professionals to guide understanding and practice and policy-related decisions.

- The literature review and synthesis process are not new to 20th- and 21st-century researchers, and in fact have a long history and evolution. There are now many different types of literature reviews and syntheses and rapidly increasing numbers of literature review and syntheses publications that are rapidly changing the field.

- The types and characteristics of literature reviews and syntheses have been categorized in different ways by expert reviewers. These approaches are suited to answer diverse questions in relation to using literature review and synthesis processes

- In this text, the term *literature synthesis* refers to the process of obtaining information from multiple sources, evaluating the information ascertained, and combining this information to inform unique and novel ways of understanding. The term *literature review* refers to a process whereby the reviewer examines the relevant literature on a chosen topic, on a limited to an expansive spectrum. Terms closely related to literature review and literature synthesis include evidence synthesis, research synthesis, systematic review, meta-analysis, meta-synthesis, narrative, review, annotated bibliography, and primary and secondary research—each with distinct but related meanings.

- There are highly respected scientific resources that provide guidance regarding the steps in conducting a literature review and synthesis. These steps follow similar processes and provide the structure for completing a scientifically sound literature review and synthesis.

- Literature reviews and syntheses are conducted for multiple reasons. Literature reviews and syntheses provide different types of information that is used as part of the process to guide nurses and healthcare and health policy professionals in making decisions and determining future research and practice directions.

- Bloom's Taxonomy provides a useful framework for understanding the cognitive skills that are necessary for creating a strong literature review and synthesis, including knowledge, comprehension, application, analysis, synthesis, and evaluation.

- Multiple literature review and synthesis resources exist globally. Most of these resources are available, at least partially, to professionals worldwide, and inform expansive understanding.

REFERENCES

Aromataris, E., & Munn, Z. (2017). Chapter 1: JBI systematic reviews. In E. Aromataris & Z. Munn (Eds.) *Joanna Briggs Institute reviewer's manual*. The Joanna Briggs Institute, 2017. https://reviewersmanual.joannabriggs.org/

Aveyard, H., & Bradbury-Jones, C. (2019). An analysis of current practices in undertaking literature reviews in nursing: Findings from a focused mapping review and synthesis. *BMC Medical Research Methodology, 19*, 105. https://doi.org/10.1186/s12874-019-0751-7f

Barnes, A., & Patrick, S. (2019). Lay summaries of clinical study results: An overview. *Pharmaceutical Medicine, 33*(4), 261–268. https://doi.org/10.1007/s40290-019-00285-0

Bettany-Saltikov, J., & McSherry, R. (2016). *How to do a systematic literature review in nursing: A step-by-step guide*. Open University Press.

Bolderston, A. (2008). Writing an effective literature review. *Journal of Medical Imaging and Radiation Sciences, 39*, 86–92. https://doi.org/10.1016/j.jmir.2008.04.009

Booth, A., Sutton, A., & Papaioannou, D. (2016). *Systematic approaches to a successful literature review*. SAGE.

Brettle, A., & Gambling, T. (2003). Needle in a haystack? Effective literature searching for research. *Radiography*, 9, 229–236. https://doi.org/10.1016/S1078-8174(03)00064-6

Campbell Collaboration. (2021). *Campbell systematic reviews*. https://campbellcollaboration.org/better-evidence.html

Chalmers, I., Hedges, L. V., & Cooper, H. (2002). A brief history of research synthesis. *Evaluation & the Health Professions*, 25(1), 12–37. https://doi.org/10.1177/0163278702025001003

Clarke, M. (2018). Partially systematic thoughts on the history of systematic reviews. *Systematic Reviews*, 7(176), 1–6. https://doi.org/10.1186/s13643-018-0833-3

Clarke, M., & Chalmers, I. (2018). Reflections on the history of systematic reviews. *BMJ Evidence-Based Medicine*, 23(4). https://doi.org/10.1136/bmjebm-2018-110968

Cochrane Training. (2021). *Chapter 1: Introduction*. https://training.cochrane.org/handbook/current/chapter-i#section-i-1

Conn, V. S., & Coon Sells, T. G. (2014). Is it time to write a review article? *Western Journal of Nursing Research*, 36(4), 435–439. https://doi.org/10.1177/0193945913519060

Cooper, H. M. (1985). A Taxonomy of literature reviews. Paper Presented at the Annual Meeting of the American Educational Research Association (69th, Chicago, IL, March 31–April 4, 1985). ERIC database. https://files.eric.ed.gov/fulltext/ED254541.pdf

Cooper, H. (2017). *Research synthesis and meta-analysis: A step-by-step approach* (5th ed.). Sage.

Cooper, H., & Hedges, L. V. (2009). Research synthesis as a scientific process. In H. Cooper, L. V. Hedges, & J. C. Valentine (Eds.), *The handbook of research synthesis* (pp. 3–16). Russell Sage Foundation.

Cooper, H., Hedges, L. V., & Valentine, J. C. (Eds.) (2019). *The handbook of research synthesis and meta-analysis*. Russell Sage Foundation.

Critical Appraisal Skills Programme. (2018). *CASP critical appraisal checklists*. http://www.casp-uk.net/

Cronin, P., Ryan, F., & Coughlan, M. (2008). Undertaking a literature review: A step-by-step approach. *British Journal of Nursing (Mark Allen Publishing)*, 17(1), 38–43. https://doi.org/10.12968/bjon.2008.17.1.28059

Derish, P. A., & Annesley, T. M. (2011). How to write a rave review. *Clinical Chemistry*, 57(3), 388–391. https://doi.org/10.1373/clinchem.2010.160622

Eden, J., Levit, L., Berg, A., & Morton, S. (2011). *Finding what works in health care: Standards for systematic reviews*. Washington, D.C.: The National Academies Press.

Elliott, J. H., Synnot, A., Turner, T., Simmonds, M., Akl, E. A., McDonald, S., Salanti, G., Meerpohl, J., MacLehose, H., Hilton, J., Tovey, D., Shemilt, I., & Thomas, J. (2017). Living systematic review: 1. Introduction-the why, what, when, and how. *Journal of Clinical Epidemiology*, 91, 23–30. https://doi.org/10.1016/j.jclinepi.2017.08.010.

Fink, A. (2020). *Conducting research literature reviews* (5th ed.). SAGE.

Galvan, J. L., & Galvan, M. C. (2017). *Writing literature reviews: A guide for students of the social and behavioral sciences* (7th ed.). Routledge, Taylor & Francis Group.

Garrard, J. (2017). *Health sciences literature review made easy: The matrix method* (5th ed.). Jones & Bartlett Learning.

Gough, D., Thomas, J., & Oliver, S. (2012). Clarifying differences between review designs and methods. *Systematic Reviews*, 1, 28. https://doi.org/10.1186/2046-4053-1-28

Granello, D. H. (2001). Promoting cognitive complexity in graduate written work: Using Bloom's taxonomy as a pedagogical tool to improve literature reviews. *Counselor Education & Supervision*, 40, 292–307.

Higgins, J., & Thomas, J. (2021). *Cochrane handbook for systematic reviews of interventions, Version 62*. https://training.cochrane.org/handbook/current

Hong, Q. N., & Pluye, P. (2018). Systematic reviews: A brief historical overview. *Education for Information (Special Issue)*, 34(4), 261–276. https://doi.org/10.3233/EFI-180219

Iwuchukwu, M. O. (2015). Literature review and use of Benjamin Bloom's taxonomy. *International Journal of Humanities and Cultural Studies*, 2(3), 436–444.

Joanna Briggs Institute. (2021). *Critical appraisal tools*. https://jbi.global/critical-appraisal-tools

Johnson, R., Watkinson, A., & Mabe, M. (2018). *The STM report: An overview of scientific and scholarly publishing*. International Association of Scientific, Technical and Medical Publishers.

Khan, K., Kunz, R., Kleijnen, J., & Antes, G. (2011). *Systematic reviews to support evidence-based medicine* (2nd ed.). Hodder Arnold (Hodder Education).

Lasserson, T. J., Thomas, J., & Higgins, J. P. T. (2019). Chapter 1: Starting a review. In J. P. T. Higgins, J. Thomas, J. Chandler, M. Cumpston, T. Li, M. J. Page, & V. A. Welch (Eds.). *Cochrane handbook for systematic reviews of interventions Version 6.0*. www.training.cochrane.org/handbook

Lefebvre, C., Glanville, J., Briscoe, S., Littlewood, A., Marshall, C., Metzendorf, M. I., Noel-Storr, A., Rader, T., Shokraneh, F., Thomas, J., & Wieland, L. S. (2019). Chapter 4: Searching for and selecting studies. In J. P. T. Higgins, J. Thomas, J. Chandler, M. Cumpston, T. Li, M. J. Page, & V. A. Welch (Eds.). *Cochrane handbook for systematic reviews of interventions Version 6.0*. www.training.cochrane.org/handbook

Lewis, S., & Clarke, M. (2001). Forest plots: Trying to see the wood and the trees. *BMJ, 322*, 1479–1480.

Littell, J. H. (2018, July). Conceptual and practical classification of research reviews and other evidence synthesis products. *The Campbell Collaboration*, pp. 1–21. https://doi.org/10.4073/cmdp.2018.1

Littell, J. H., Corcoran, J., & Pillai, V. (2008). *Systematic reviews and meta-analysis*. Oxford University Press.

Liumbruno, G. M., Velati, C., Pasqualetti, P., & Franchini, M. (2013). How to write a scientific manuscript for publication. *Journal of Blood Transfusion, 11*, 217–226. https://doi.org/10.2450/2012.0247-12.

Lockwood, C., Porritt, K., Munn, Z., Rittenmeyer, L., Salmond, S., Bjerrum, M., Loveday, H., Carrier, J., & Stannard, D. (2020). Chapter 2. Systematic reviews of qualitative evidence. In E. Aromataris, & Z. Munn (Eds.). *JBI manual for evidence synthesis*. JBI. https://wiki.jbi.global/display/MANUAL/Chapter+2%3A+Systematic+reviews+of+qualitative+evidence

Mahood, Q., Van Eerd, D., & Irvin, E. (2014). Searching for grey literature for systematic reviews challenges and benefits. *Research Synthesis Methods, 5*(3), 221–234. https://doi.org/10.1002/jrsm.1106

McArthur, A., Klugarova, J., Yan, H., & Florescu, S. (2020). Chapter 4: Systematic reviews of text and opinion. In E. Aromataris & Z. Munn (Eds.). *JBI manual for evidence synthesis*. JBI. https://wiki.jbi.global/display/MANUAL/Chapter+4%3A+Systematic+reviews+of+text+and+opinion

McKenzie, J. E., Brennan, S. E., Ryan, R. E., Thomson, H. J., & Johnston, R. V. (2019). Chapter 9: Summarizing study characteristics and preparing for synthesis. In J. P. T. Higgins, J. Thomas, J. Chandler, M. Cumpston, T. Li, M. J. Page, & V. A. Welch (Eds.). *Cochrane handbook for systematic reviews of interventions Version 6.0*. www.training.cochrane.org/handbook

Mlinaric, A., Horvat, M., & Supak Smolcic, V. (2017). Dealing with the positive publication bias: Why you should really publish your negative results. *Biochemia Medica, 27*(3), 030201. https://doi.org/10.11613/BM.2017.030201

Moola, S., Munn, Z., Tufanaru, C., Aromataris, E., Sears, K., Sfetcu, R., Currie, M., Lisy, K., Qureshi, R., Mattis, P., & Mu, P. (2017). Chapter 7: Systematic reviews of etiology and risk. In E. Aromataris & Z. Munn (Eds.). *JBI manual for evidence synthesis*. JBI. https://wiki.jbi.global/display/MANUAL/Chapter+7%3A+Systematic+reviews+of+etiology+and+risk

National Library of Medicine. (2021). *PubMed help*. https://pubmed.ncbi.nlm.nih.gov/#:~:text=PubMed%C2%AE%20comprises%20more%20than,science%20journals%2C%20and%20online%20books

Noyes, J., Booth, A., Cargo, M., Flemming, K., Harden, A., Harris, J., Garside, R., Hannes, K., Pantoja, T., & Thomas, J. (2019). Chapter 21: Qualitative evidence. In J. P. T. Higgins, J. Thomas, J. Chandler, M. Cumpston, T. Li, M. J. Page, & V. A. Welch (Eds.), *Cochrane handbook for systematic reviews of interventions Version 6.0*. www.training.cochrane.org/handbook

Pautasso, M. (2013). Ten simple rules for writing a literature review. *PLOS Computational Biology, 9*(7), e1003149. https://doi.org/10.1371/journal.pcbi.1003149.g001

PCORI [Patient-Centered Outcomes Research Institute]. (2019). *Evidence synthesis*. https://www.pcori.org/research-results/evidence-synthesis

Pedhazur, E. J., & Schmelkin, L. P. (1991). *Measurement, design, and analysis: An integrated approach*. Taylor & Francis.

Pericic, T. P., & Tanveer, S. (2019, July). *Why systematic reviews matter: A brief history, overview and practical guide for authors*. https://www.elsevier.com/connect/authors-update/why-systematic-reviews-matter

Petticrew, M., & Roberts, H. (2006). *Systematic reviews in the social sciences: A practical guide*. Blackwell.

PROSPERO. (2019). *International prospective register of systematic reviews*. https://www.crd.york.ac.uk/PROSPERO/

Schick-Makaroff, K., MacDonald, M., Plummer, M., Burgess, J., & Neander, W. (2016). What synthesis methodology should I use? A review and analysis of approaches to research synthesis. *AIMS Public Health, 3*(1), 172–215. https://doi.org/10.3934/publichealth.2016.1.172

Shellenbarger, T. (2016). Simplifying synthesis. *Nurse Author & Editor, 26*(3), 3.

Thomas, J., Kneale, D., McKenzie, J. E., Brennan, S. E., & Bhaumik, S. (2019). Chapter 2: Determining the scope of the review and the questions it will address. In J. P. T. Higgins, J. Thomas, J. Chandler, M. Cumpston, T. Li, M. J. Page, & V. A. Welch (Eds.). *Cochrane handbook for systematic reviews of interventions Version 6.0.* www.training.cochrane.org/handbook

Timmins, F., & McCabe, C. (2005). How to conduct an effective literature search. *Nursing Standard, 20*(1), 41–47.

Tricco, A. C., Zarin, W., Rios, P., Nincic, V., Khan, P. A., Ghassemi, M., Diaz, S., Pham, B., Straus, S. E., & Langlois, E. V. (2018). Engaging policy-makers, health system managers, and policy analysts in the knowledge synthesis process: A scoping review. *Implementation Science, 13*(1), 31. https://doi.org/10.1186/s13012-018-0717-x

Torraco, R. J. (2005). Writing integrative literature reviews: Guidelines and examples. *Human Resource Development Review, 4*(3), 356–367. https://doi.org/10.1177/1534484305278283

Tufanaru, C., Munn, Z., Aromataris, E., Campbell, J., & Hopp, L. (2020) Chapter 3: Systematic reviews of effectiveness. In E. Aromataris, & Z. Munn (Eds.). *JBI manual for evidence synthesis.* JBI. https://wiki.jbi.global/display/MANUAL/Chapter+3%3A+Systematic+reviews+of+effectiveness

Whittemore, R. (2005). Combining evidence in nursing research: Methods and implications. *Nursing Research, 54*(1), 56–62.

2

Literature Review and Synthesis Typology

Susan W. Buchholz and Kirsten A. Dickins

With the increasing recognition, acceptance, and demand for literature reviews has come a rapid expansion in the methodological approaches available, as well as a proliferation in the language used to describe these varied approaches to literature reviews.

CHAPTER OUTLINE

- Objectives
- Differentiating Between the Multiple Types of Literature Reviews and Syntheses
- Similarities and Differences Between the Types of Literature Reviews and Syntheses
- Determining When a Literature Review and Synthesis is Needed
- Typology of Selected Literature Reviews and Syntheses
- Selecting a Type of Literature Review and Synthesis
- Activities
- Summary Points
- References

This chapter provides an overview of different types of literature reviews and syntheses. Although definitions continue to be refined, there is general agreement regarding a collection of unique features that define each of the different types of reviews. There are a multitude of types of literature reviews and syntheses, therefore it is not feasible to present an exhaustive list. However, we present an overview of the features, advantages, and challenges of different approaches to literature reviews and syntheses that nurses and other healthcare and health policy professionals will find useful. These approaches include critical reviews, historical reviews, integrative reviews, mapping reviews, meta-analyses, mixed methods reviews, narrative reviews, qualitative reviews, rapid reviews, realist reviews, scoping reviews, state-of-the-art reviews, systematic reviews, and umbrella reviews. As it can be challenging to determine which type of literature review and synthesis to conduct, questions are provided to help guide you toward choosing the most appropriate type of literature review and synthesis for your purpose and question.

LEARNING OBJECTIVES

This chapter contains an overview of the multiple types of literature reviews and syntheses commonly used by nurses and other healthcare professionals. By the end of this chapter, you will be able to:

- Differentiate between the multiple types of literature reviews and syntheses

- Appreciate similarities and differences between the types of literature reviews and syntheses

- Determine when a literature review and synthesis is needed

- Understand the unique purpose of each type of literature review and synthesis

- Describe how to select the correct type of literature review and synthesis

DIFFERENTIATING BETWEEN THE MULTIPLE TYPES OF LITERATURE REVIEWS AND SYNTHESES

Literature reviews have been considered a rigorous and acceptable research method for over three decades; interest in reviewing and synthesizing the literature on complex questions continues to rise among nurses and other healthcare professionals (Boland et al., 2017; Wong et al., 2013). With the increasing recognition, acceptance, and demand for literature reviews has come a rapid expansion in the methodological approaches available, as well as a proliferation in the language used to describe these varied approaches to literature reviews. Over three dozen separate terms have been associated with literature review and synthesis approaches; however, these terms are often used inconsistently, with some describing well-established literature review methods and others referring to lesser detailed methods (Aromataris & Munn, 2020a; Aveyard & Bradbury-Jones, 2019; Centre for Reviews and Dissemination, University of York, 2009; Cochrane Library, 2021; Conn & Coon Sells, 2014a; Noble & Smith, 2018; Samnani et al., 2017). While the growth of choices for literature review methods has allowed for greater precision in literature review and synthesis processes, term proliferation has also led to confusion among nurses and other healthcare students and professionals alike. Novice reviewers are often uncertain of the features, advantages, and challenges associated with each type of literature review and synthesis. This confusion may stem from lack of conceptual clarity (Aveyard & Bradbury-Jones, 2019), which threatens the capacity of literature reviews and syntheses to actualize their full potential (Samnani et al., 2017). Moreover, few types of literature reviews currently have a unified and singularly prescribed method, and many of the literature review types are not mutually exclusive, further contributing to categorical confusion (Grant & Booth, 2009).

Just as a craftsperson benefits from a keen awareness of each tool available in their toolbox, the context for the use of each tool, and the strengths and weaknesses of each tool, a reviewer is advantaged by their knowledge of the spectrum of approaches to conducting a literature review and synthesis. However, many who work with literature reviews experience obstacles to familiarity with and mastery of knowledge of research methodology and statistics (Grant & Booth, 2009). We aim in this chapter to reduce barriers to building knowledge regarding the multiple types of literature reviews and syntheses. In this chapter, we define and differentiate the multiple types of literature reviews and syntheses, highlighting the names used to label each review type, definition, purpose, features, advantages, and disadvantages, as well as the similarities across the review types. Knowing your options and the unique features of each literature review and synthesis approach will guide you in making a sound methodological decision.

SIMILARITIES AND DIFFERENCES BETWEEN THE TYPES OF LITERATURE REVIEWS AND SYNTHESES

While the method underlying each type of review is characterized by a distinct definition, purpose, sampling frame, and analysis type (Whittemore, 2005), many of the types of literature reviews and syntheses share common features. The depths reached by a reviewer at different stages of a literature review is in part dependent on the type of literature review selected, as well as the level of rigor of the approach used to follow the basics principles of the literature review type. It is incumbent upon the reviewer to carefully study the parameters of the review type to avoid labeling it as a certain type of review, when in fact it may not meet the criteria of the proclaimed type of literature review.

Reviewers generally follow a similar process when completing a literature review and synthesis. Shared features of literature reviews include identification of central issues in a topic area (Russell, 2005). An identified gap in the literature should be documented to justify why a literature review needs to be conducted. Strengths and weaknesses of existing literature regarding the topic or question are typically evaluated. Once the literature has been selected that will be included in the review, the reviewer will extract data from the literature sources. After data extraction, the reviewer will synthesize the literature findings. A completed literature review and synthesis should generate new knowledge about the selected topic. Also, literature reviews often identify gaps in current research and make future research recommendations (Russell, 2005), as well as share implications for clinical practice and policy.

DETERMINING WHEN A LITERATURE REVIEW AND SYNTHESIS IS NEEDED

Orienting yourself to the landscape of knowledge is imperative to determining your next actions. When only a handful of primary studies and only a few literature reviews are published on your topic, it is first necessary to firmly identify research questions.

You may determine that there is insufficient literature to conduct a literature review and synthesis and may need to either change your review purpose or question and place your efforts on adding primary research studies to the healthcare literature. When more primary studies but fewer literature reviews are published, you may realize that a literature review may be justifiable. It will be important to determine if a similar literature review has recently been completed and published on your intended review purpose and question. When a few primary studies and many literature reviews are published, it is necessary to raise awareness of the need for more primary studies. In this case, you may choose to contribute instead by conducting a primary research study, rather than a literature review and synthesis. When many primary studies and many literature reviews are published on a topic, you might consider conducting a review of reviews (e.g., umbrella review) to synthesize the existing literature reviews (Pautasso, 2013).

TYPOLOGY OF SELECTED LITERATURE REVIEWS AND SYNTHESES

In this section on defining different types of literature reviews and syntheses, we first showcase how three global organizations: Centre for Reviews and Dissemination, Cochrane Library, and Joanna Briggs Institute present terminology on the types of literature reviews (Boxes 2.1–2.3). These three global literature review organizations provide a typology of the multiple types of literature reviews, using systematic review

---

BOX 2.1   ORGANIZATION OF REVIEW TYPES BY THE CENTRE FOR REVIEWS AND DISSEMINATION, UNIVERSITY OF YORK (2009)

- Systematic reviews of clinical tests
- Systematic reviews of public health interventions
- Systematic reviews of adverse effects
- Systematic reviews of economic evaluation
- Incorporating qualitative evidence in or alongside effectiveness reviews

---

BOX 2.2   ORGANIZATION OF SYSTEMATIC REVIEWS BY COCHRANE LIBRARY (2021)

- Intervention reviews
- Diagnostic test accuracy reviews
- Methodology reviews
- Qualitative reviews
- Prognosis reviews

BOX 2.3   ORGANIZATION OF REVIEWS BY THE JOANNA BRIGGS INSTITUTE (AROMATARIS & MUNN, 2020b)

- Systematic reviews of qualitative evidence
- Systematic reviews of effectiveness
- Systematic reviews of text and opinion
- Systematic reviews of prevalence and incidence
- Systematic reviews of economic evidence
- Systematic reviews of etiology and risk
- Systematic reviews of measurement properties
- Mixed methods systematic reviews
- Diagnostic test accuracy systematic reviews
- Umbrella reviews
- Scoping reviews

---

criteria as the gold standard for the highest level of rigor for reviews. Regarding systematic reviews, it is useful to note that a literature review may follow systematic review principles, even if the term used to describe the review does not use the precise terminology: "systematic review." For example, a qualitative review may be a systematic review, if systematic review principles have been followed. But the term "systematic review" is not seen as part of the overarching term (e.g., qualitative systematic review). It is also helpful to remember that while a systematic process is required for a systematic review, using a systematic process does not necessarily mean that a reviewer has conducted a systematic review, per se.

There are similarities and differences in what types of reviews instructions are provided for and how these review types are named by leading organizations. As noted in Boxes 2.1 to 2.3, when comparing typologies offered by these organizations, there is variance as well as overlap in reporting of similar types of literature reviews.

In this chapter, we provide an overview of 14 types of approaches (Box 2.4) to conducting a literature review and syntheses. This is not an exhaustive list of all available types of literature reviews. There is not one globally accepted list of types of literature reviews, and interpretation of the definitions of the multiple review types continues to vary across organizations and publications. However, we have aimed to capture widely used types and definitions of literature reviews and syntheses used by nurses and other healthcare professionals. We have also sought to provide information on types of reviews that clinicians will find useful in practice arenas. While we provide a cursory overview of different literature review and synthesis types, we encourage you to go beyond these overviews to dive deeper into the resources dedicated to the literature review and synthesis types that are most appropriate to your review purpose and

---

BOX 2.4   LITERATURE REVIEW TYPOLOGY

1. Critical Reviews
2. Historical Reviews
3. Integrative Reviews
4. Mapping Reviews
5. Meta-Analyses
6. Mixed Methods Reviews
7. Narrative Reviews
8. Qualitative Reviews
9. Rapid Reviews
10. Realist Reviews
11. Scoping Reviews
12. State-of-the-Art Reviews
13. Systematic Reviews
14. Umbrella Reviews

---

question. For organizational ease, we present types of literature review and synthesis in alphabetical order, which is not a reflection of their relative importance.

Critical Review

[Other name: Narrative Critical Review]
A critical review is designed to present, analyze, and synthesize material from diverse data sources, and incorporate assessment of the strengths, weaknesses, and validity of the cited resources. A critical review can tell a story about what is already known to provide a platform for advancing knowledge on a selected topic. A critical review of the current research can also be completed before designing and executing primary studies on a selected topic or conducting a more extensive literature review (Grant & Booth, 2009; Jesson & Lacey, 2006; Samnani et al., 2017). A unique feature of the critical review is the emphasis on the incorporation of different and competing schools of thought on a topic. A critical review may provide a model that results from the synthesis of existing models or different schools of thought. Alternatively, or additionally, a critical review may provide an entirely new interpretation of the existing data with a unique idea on an existing topic, a new school of thought, or generation of a new hypothesis (Grant & Booth, 2009; Samnani et al., 2017).

Advantages

The advantages of the critical review include the identification and evaluation of the value of the current body of literature on a given topic as well as recognition of experts in a subject area. This evaluation allows the reader to make judgments about the topic of interest, and ideally, be able to distinguish between facts and opinions on a subject (Grant & Booth, 2009; Samnani et al., 2017; Saunders & Rojon, 2011). A critical review can serve as a springboard for the next phase of conceptual development and testing and can also be used to provide a resolution on competing viewpoints.

Challenges

A critical review may demonstrate a lower level or a lack of systematicity, in part depending on how rigorously the reviewers undertake the critical review process. In the event that systematicity is reduced, then bias may be present in the results (Grant & Booth, 2009; Samnani et al., 2017).

Exemplar

The following critical review examines the current literature on rates and reasons for hospital admissions from nursing homes. The authors use original research articles as well as literature reviews. The authors conclude the critical review by noting that there were many similar research designs and few alternatives in relation to study design. The authors suggest that a focus on potential hospitalizations would add to the overall understanding, that the everyday practice should be further studied, and that the work could be analyzed at a more in-depth level.

- Agotnes, G., Jacobsen, F. F., & Harrington, C. Petersen, K. A. (2016). A critical review of research on hospitalization from nursing homes: What is missing? *Ageing International, 41*, 3–16. https://doi.org/10.1007/s12126-015-9232-4

  www.link.springer.com/content/pdf/10.1007%2Fs12126-015-9232-4.pdf

Historical Review

The temporal component of a specific topic is the main focus of a historical review. The reviewer outlines the chronological timeline of the development of a topic, to describe how it has changed or remained stable over time. For instance, shifts in how a health condition is viewed by the healthcare workforce and the public over a specified time period might be detailed in a historical review. Significant points in time are established, which have influenced the findings in the care of individuals that are affected by specific health conditions. This includes changes not only in diagnosis and treatment but also theoretical and methodological changes that influence healthcare management (Conn & Coon Sells, 2014a).

Advantages

In a historical review, the perspective given to a selected topic occurs by placing it within the context of time (Hart, 2018). The reviewer can document what was known at the start of a specified period of time, and how knowledge shifted or changed over time, including the theoretical components and phenomena that emerged along with the topic. This historical snapshot can provide a foundation for identifying future research directions.

Challenges

A historical review may require additional training on how to conduct historical analyses. Also, if the reviewer does not obtain comprehensive information on historical events—either because this information is difficult to locate or missed because a certain database was not searched—the reviewer could overlook important contributions to the developmental timeline of the topic.

Exemplar

While there are many examples of how views, research, and treatment approaches to specific disease processes have changed over time, perhaps one of the most salient illustrations is that of the human immunodeficiency virus (HIV). The following is an exemplar of a historical review, with a specific focus on the construction of a timeline of HIV interventions in British Columbia, Canada.

- Olding, M., Enns, B., Panagiotoglou, D., Shoveller, J., Harrigan, P. R., Barrios, R., Kerr, T., Montaner, J. S. G., & Nosyk, B. (2017). A historical review of HIV prevention and care initiatives in British Columbia, Canada: 1996 to 2015. *Journal of the International AIDS Society, 20*(1), 21941. https://doi.org/10.7448/IAS.20.1.21941

  www.ncbi.nlm.nih.gov/pmc/articles/PMC5640311/pdf/jias-20-1371937.pdf

Integrative Review

[Other names: Integrative Synthesis; Integrative Literature Review; Integrative Research Review]

The purpose of an integrative review is to review, critique, and synthesize varied types of literature on a selected topic, allowing for the generation of new frameworks and perspectives (Torraco, 2016). An integrative review is generally conducted on a dynamic topic on which literature has rapidly grown and has not undergone a comprehensive review and update over an extended time period. The sampling frame of an integrative review allows for inclusion of articles with diverse methodological approaches, including empirical (quantitative; qualitative; mixed methods; randomized controlled trials; longitudinal studies; retrospective studies; cross-sectional studies), methodological (designs; methods; analyses), and theoretical literature (including both supporting and non-supporting literature) (Russell, 2005). The ability to incorporate diverse methodologies provides the reviewer with an opportunity to use multiple data sources to inform the synthesis process (Whittemore & Knafl, 2005). Further, an integrative review can extend beyond the examination of research findings, to provide a theoretical review and/or platform for concept development.

Advantages

In an integrative review, the reviewer can bridge gaps between related areas of work, allowing for greater depth and breadth of conclusions drawn (Russell, 2005), creating a comprehensive picture of a given topic (Whittemore & Knafl, 2005). Another strength of the integrative review is its utility in exploring and determining which research methods have been successfully used to investigate a certain topic. An integrative review is also useful in identifying and synthesizing an explanation of theoretical or conceptual frameworks (Russell, 2005).

Challenges

When conducting an integrative review, it can often be challenging to combine data from studies using different designs and methodological approaches; thus, a sophisticated integrative review analysis can be complicated and may require special training (Russell, 2005). Depending on the purpose and approach taken by the reviewer, an integrative review may have imbedded bias, especially if lacking in procedural rigor.

Exemplar

The following integrative review examines maternal engagement within the setting of the neonatal intensive care unit (NICU), relating maternal engagement to health outcomes of mothers and infants alike. The reviewers do not limit their search to a specific methodology, including studies using multiple methodologies to measure maternal engagement activities. They assess infant outcomes and maternal health–behavior outcomes. In their results, the reviewers report the findings of the review as categorized by study design.

- Klawetter, S., Greenfield, J. C., Speer, S. R., Brown, K., & Hwang, S. S. (2019). An integrative review: Maternal engagement in the neonatal intensive care unit and health outcomes for U.S.-born preterm infants and their parents. *AIMS Public Health*, 6(2), 160–183. https://doi.org/10.3934/publichealth.2019.2.160

  www.ncbi.nlm.nih.gov/pmc/articles/PMC6606523/pdf/publichealth-06-02-160.pdf

Mapping Review

[Other names: Systematic Map; Focused Mapping Review and Synthesis]
A mapping review is focused on classifying, or "mapping," trends and categorizing existing literature on a selected topic (Aveyard & Bradbury-Jones, 2019; Grant & Booth, 2009). The purpose of a mapping review is to identify evidence gaps and suggest new topics or directions for either primary studies or a more rigorous literature review (Grant & Booth, 2009; Samnani et al., 2017). A mapping review can categorize studies according to the reviewer's discretion and may characterize studies in various ways; for example, by theoretical perspective, population group, or study setting.

Advantages

A mapping review can contextualize literature within the broader evidence base. A mapping review can provide the foundation to make an informed decision regarding whether the available studies can answer a review question, and if so, whether to undertake an in-depth review and synthesis on all or a subset of studies (Grant & Booth, 2009). Further, a mapping review can reveal whether the totality of studies is sufficiently similar for a coherent, robust synthesis. Importantly, a mapping review can offer decision-makers (e.g., clinicians, researchers, policymakers) an explicit and transparent means of identifying practice- and policy-relevant review questions (Grant & Booth, 2009; Samnani et al., 2017).

Challenges

A mapping review often places less emphasis on analysis and synthesis, in comparison to other literature review types. Broad descriptions of studies may oversimplify the picture or mask variation (heterogeneity) across study findings, though this in part depends on the degree of detail sought and conveyed by the reviewer. Studies included in a mapping review are typically characterized on design and may not have an in-depth quality assessment (Grant & Booth, 2009).

Exemplar

The following mapping review addresses the conduct of research and knowledge creation regarding children and youth in Greenland over 40 years. The reviewers list each study and then identify characteristics of the research methods used and themes derived within each respective study. After synthesizing the different studies, the reviewers recommend that individuals completing literature reviews use more qualitative, locally grounded approaches in their studies addressing issues relevant to youth in Greenland.

- Glendøs, M., & Berline, P. (2017). Forty years of research concerning children and youth in Greenland: A mapping review. *International Journal of Circumpolar Health*, *76*(1), 1–13. https://doi.org/10.1080/22423982.2017.1323526.

  www.ncbi.nlm.nih.gov/pmc/articles/PMC5497539/pdf/zich-76-1323526.pdf

Meta-Analysis

A meta-analysis refers to the outcome of using standardized statistical procedures to combine, analyze, and summarize quantitative findings from multiple primary studies. The purpose of a meta-analysis is to integrate quantitative findings from several studies with related or identical hypotheses to transform the results into a common metric. A meta-analysis calculates a more precise aggregated, overall effect, effect magnitude, and subsample effects (Biondi-Zoccai, 2016; Cronin et al., 2008; Grant & Booth, 2009; Moher et al., 2015; Samnani et al., 2017; Whittemore, 2005). While a meta-analysis can be performed on as few as two studies, generally a meta-analysis aims for an exhaustive and comprehensive identification and inclusion of all relevant and related studies (Grant & Booth, 2009; Littell et al., 2008; Samnani et al., 2017). Studies included in a meta-analysis must be sufficiently similar to ensure validity; outcomes must be similar, measured in the same or similar ways, and be within the same or similar time interval. A meta-analysis most commonly accompanies a systematic review.

Advantages

The statistical techniques of a meta-analysis leverage data from individual studies that are independently insufficient to impact practice and policy; data are assimilated into a composite evidence base that provides more precise estimates of effects when considered altogether (Grant & Booth, 2009; Moher et al., 2015). Moreover, large datasets can be placed into figures and tables that provide a quick summary for the reader, which are efficient evidence-based references for decision-makers (Grant & Booth, 2009).

Challenges

The major disadvantage of a meta-analysis is the inability to compensate for sub-optimal design quality of the included primary studies. Additionally, a meta-analysis may attempt to incorporate disparate or insufficiently similar primary study designs (Grant & Booth, 2009; Samnani et al., 2017). The execution of a meta-analysis may require considerable time, special software, and extensive knowledge. It is beneficial for a reviewer to be on a team that contains the experience and resources required to appropriately execute and complete a meta-analysis.

Exemplar

The following meta-analysis included over 700 trials and was executed in tandem with a systematic review investigating the outcomes of medication adherence interventions. The reviewers used meta-analytic moderator analyses to examine associations between different aspects of medication adherence, including effect sizes for adherence, and characteristics of the sample, design and intervention. Their multiple analyses suggested that medication adherence would more likely improve, if health careproviders used behavioral strategies instead of cognitive strategies.

- Conn, V. S., & Ruppar, T. M. (2017). Medication adherence outcomes of 771 intervention trials: Systematic review and meta-analysis. *Preventive Medicine, 99*, 269–276. https://doi.org/10.1016/j.ypmed.2017.03.008.

  www.ncbi.nlm.nih.gov/pmc/articles/PMC5467216/pdf/nihms862780.pdf

Mixed Methods Review

[Other name: Mixed Studies Review]
A mixed methods review integrates both quantitative and qualitative primary studies. A variety of approaches can be used to conduct a mixed methods review, and different

terminology is used to describe the process of a mixed methods review (Pearson, 2015; Sandelowski et al., 2006). Given that knowledge, here we provide an introduction to three types of processes that can be used in a mixed methods review. In a *segregated approach*, reviewers initially examine and synthesize studies with methods appropriate to the type of methodology initially used in the quantitative and qualitative studies. After separate syntheses, the results from the quantitative and qualitative studies are then brought together to be synthesized. In a *linked approach*, quantitative and qualitative data sources may interface at multiple points throughout the review process, and the quantitative and qualitative data can be directly compared, but not merged together. In an *integration approach*, quantitative and qualitative data are assimilated at the outset. Through this mixed methods data integration, quantitative data can be converted into qualitative data, and qualitative data can be converted into quantitative data. While there are different configurations to using an integration approach, a widely respected method translates the data obtained from an initial quantitative synthesis into qualitative data. These transformed data are then pooled with initial qualitative synthesis findings. Whichever approach is selected, or how it is named, it is vital for the reviewer to justify the decision to undertake a mixed methods review and use the chosen approach.

Advantages

There are multiple advantages to conducting a mixed methods review. A mixed methods review provides an opportunity for reviewers to examine phenomena of interest more comprehensively by integrating both quantitative and qualitative data. Mixed methods research can provide guidance on explaining unexpected findings from both quantitative and qualitative perspectives (Doyle et al., 2016), as qualitative methods can address shortcomings in an explanation of quantitative methods, while quantitative data can numerically and precisely explain a phenomenon not quantified by qualitative approaches. Altogether, a mixed methods review allows decision-makers to arrive at a more complete understanding of a particular condition or intervention (Grant & Booth, 2009).

Challenges

The methodological challenges of appraising and synthesizing both quantitative and qualitative research in the setting of a mixed methods review can be overwhelming for a novice reviewer. These methodological challenges relate to considering a range of designs that address different though related questions and were conducted under distinct research paradigms (Grant & Booth, 2009). Further, there is no one agreed upon approach to the synthesis of the literature in a mixed methods review (Doyle et al., 2016; Pearson et al., 2015; Sandelowski, 2014). Given the number of different approaches that a reviewer can take to conducting a mixed methods review, the reviewer who is new to this method will require the resources of a team including an experienced mixed methods reviewer. A new reviewer should also take into consideration that they will likely need the resources for mixed methods review training.

Exemplar

The following mixed methods review examined nutrition-related social media use in young adults. In this mixed methods review, using a segregated approach, the authors use the findings from the qualitative studies to provide a narrative explanation for the findings derived from the quantitative analysis. The reviewers note that concerns young adults have regarding social media use can impact engagement when taking part in research that aims to influence weight. Thus, reviewers call for a need to determine more effective methods to use social media to promote healthy choices.

- Klassen, K. M., Douglass, C. H., Brennan, L., Truby, H., & Lim, M. S. C. (2018). Social media use for nutrition outcomes in young adults: A mixed-methods systematic review. *The International Journal of Behavioral Nutrition and Physical Activity, 15*(1), 70-018-0696-y. https://doi.org/10.1186/s12966-018-0696-y

  www.ncbi.nlm.nih.gov/pmc/articles/PMC6057054/pdf/12966_2018_Article_696.pdf

Narrative Review

[Other names: Narrative Overview; Scholarly Review; Structured Narrative Review; Unsystematic/Non-Systematic Narrative Review]

The narrative review is one of the broadest types of literature reviews. The term "narrative review" typically holds a more general meaning and often provides an overview or broad perspective on a given topic area. There is no consensus on the standard structure of a narrative review. A published narrative review generally follows the preferred format of the journal in which it appears (Ferrari, 2015). A narrative review responds to an unanswered question(s) by describing and/or appraising published articles on a selected topic (Cronin et al., 2008; Ferrari, 2015). A narrative review may include certain features of a systematic review (e.g., literature selection flow chart; Ferrari, 2015). A reviewer may see considerable variance across narrative reviews; a methods section, including eligibility criteria, may or may not be explicitly specified in a narrative review. Additionally, a narrative review may only include literature sources from one singular database, although a narrative review can also include sources from multiple databases.

Advantages

A narrative review can include non-empirical literature, such as editorials and commentaries. Further, a narrative review can stand alone or may be part of a larger literature review, emphasizing differing degrees of systematicity. A narrative review can provide an overview of a topic area, which may be valuable for those who are initially familiarizing themselves with a topic area (Grant & Booth, 2009). Additionally, a narrative review can help to track a thread of development of a scientific principle or clinical concept, which may be lost in a systematic review due to often more strict criteria (Ferrari, 2015). While some researchers use narrative review findings as part of a background of another manuscript, others may publish a narrative review as a stand-alone manuscript.

Challenges

It can often be difficult to replicate a narrative review (Ferrari, 2015; Smith & Noble, 2016), as the reviewers may not have followed a systematic process. A narrative review also may only include, analyze, and synthesize a small sample of primary studies. Additionally, if the studies reviewed represent only a subset of a larger group of similar studies, the study findings may be biased (Smith & Noble, 2016). Narrative reviews may be difficult to publish if the reviewer limits the number of databases searched.

Exemplar

The following narrative review addresses the burden of migraine headaches. The reviewers searched one database, using a relatively stream-lined search strategy. Major themes and main results are descriptively reported.

- Leonardi, M., & Raggi, A. (2019). A narrative review on the burden of migraine: When the burden is the impact on people's life. *The Journal of Headache and Pain*, *20*(1), 41-019–0993-0. https://doi.org/10.1186/s10194-019-0993-0

  www.thejournalofheadacheandpain.biomedcentral.com/track/pdf/10.1186/s10194-019-0993-0

Qualitative Review

A qualitative review considers, compares, and synthesizes qualitative (or non-numeric) studies. Historically, a qualitative review has been understood as the summarization of studies, but not the statistical combination thereof (Grant & Booth, 2009). The purpose of a qualitative review is to identify concepts, metaphors, and/or themes that exist within or across individual qualitative studies, which comprise the units of study (Lockwood et al., 2020). A qualitative review may inform research and/or clinical practice, primarily by summarizing processes or experiences (Whittemore, 2005). Qualitative methodologies used in primary studies may include discourse analysis, ethnography, feminist research, grounded theory, participatory action research, and phenomenology, among others. Qualitative data reported in the primary studies may be generated from a variety of sources, including individual interviews, focus groups, fieldwork notes, and/or journaling (Lockwood et al., 2020). There are distinct synthesis methods recommended by different organizations and qualitative reviewers, including but not limited to meta-aggregation, meta-ethnography, thematic analysis/synthesis, grounded theory, narrative synthesis, meta-study, and meta-summary synthesis (Barnett-Page & Thomas, 2009; Centre for Reviews and Dissemination, University of York, 2009; Lockwood et al., 2020).

Advantages

A qualitative review has strong potential for the development of a new theory, an overarching narrative, or a wider generalization. Use of qualitative methods is increasing within evidence-based healthcare research, thus there is a rising abundance of rich qualitative data; using these data to inform qualitative reviews allows readers to understand perceptions of health from the individual and community level, by familiarizing policy and other decision-makers about patient healthcare experiences (Lockwood et al., 2020). In other words, a qualitative review may be particularly helpful, as aggregated and synthesized findings from multiple primary qualitative studies may be more powerful than isolated comments from local questionnaires, surveys (Grant & Booth, 2009), individual interviews, focus groups, fieldwork notes, or journals.

Challenges

Although the qualitative review has become more popular in the published literature, not all reviewers have adequate experience or knowledge to conduct a qualitative review. A qualitative review requires additional training, and typically a novice qualitative reviewer will need to work with experts in qualitative methodologies (Grant & Booth, 2009) or receive training in the synthesis of qualitative studies (Lockwood et al., 2020). It may also be challenging to locate a sufficient number of studies that use the same or similar qualitative methodology, which may render it difficult to draw equitable comparisons across findings and may require additional synthesis skills on the part of the reviewer.

Exemplar

In the following qualitative review, the reviewers explore the beliefs, expectations, and values of women during childbirth. However, there were a wide range of designs of the 35 included studies (e.g., phenomenological interviews, focus groups). The authors used the Noblitt and Harre (1988) method to analyze the data, which is based on constant comparison. This qualitative review helped to inform the World Health Organization (WHO) intrapartum guidelines.

- Downe, S., Finlayson, K., Oladapo, O. T., Bonet, M., & Gulmezoglu, A. M. (2018). What matters to women during childbirth: A systematic qualitative review. *PLOS One, 13*(4), e0194906. https://doi.org/10.1371/journal.pone.0194906

  www.ncbi.nlm.nih.gov/pmc/articles/PMC5903648/pdf/pone.0194906.pdf

Rapid Review

[Other name: Rapid Evidence Assessment]
A rapid review is a succinct review type aiming to provide concise information on a selected topic in an expedited fashion. In a rapid review, the steps of a systematic review are streamlined (Biondi-Zoccai, 2016; Noble & Smith, 2018; Tricco et al., 2017). A rapid review is typically intended to provide interim guidance on a topic until resources are available to conduct a more rigorous review (Hailey et al., 2000; Watt et al., 2008).

The reviewer often chooses which stages of the review to limit and must then explicitly project and report the likely effect of such limitations. Reviewers should also be sure to document the methodology used to reduce bias (Grant & Booth, 2009), especially in light of the stated limitations. To shorten the review timeframe, reviewers can narrowly focus the review purpose and question; limit the number of databases searched, including restricting the amount of grey literature screened; extract only key variables; perform single screening of full-texts instead of dual screening of titles/abstracts and full-texts; and perform only an abbreviated versus extensive quality appraisal of included data sources (Grant & Booth, 2009; Patnode et al., 2018). While there are recognized strategies to expedite the review, it is important that the features of a streamlined approach are both pre-specified by the review team and retain sound scientific review principles (Patnode et al., 2018).

Advantages

When timeframes are shortened or intentionally restricted, hand searching relevant reference lists for references addressing a certain purpose or question can often be effective in a rapid review, as long as consultation with content experts regarding key articles occurs (Royle & Waugh, 2003). Rapidly reviewing the literature can provide relevant evidence and actionable recommendations in a timely and cost-effective manner (Tricco et al., 2017) and avoid the increased time and resource cost associated with more structured, rigorous review types (Topfer et al., 1999).

Challenges

A rapid review may potentially omit detail regarding the methods employed in the review and may not report the projected implications of rapid review methods with respect to potential bias (Ganann et al., 2010). The reviewer must demonstrate an understanding of the implications of what is lost in the costs of lack of rigor versus the benefit of producing the evidence within a rapid timeframe (Ganann et al., 2010; Grant & Booth, 2009). Fast-tracking the methods, thereby accelerating the search and data extraction processes, may lead to overlooking relevant information and studies, including both published and grey literature (Ganann et al., 2010; Noble & Smith, 2018). Limiting critical appraisal or quality assessment may result in disproportionate inclusion of poorer quality research. Relatedly, a limited or incomplete synthesis may miss inconsistencies or contradictions in the included literature. While a rapid review may serve a particular purpose or answer a certain question pertaining to particular settings or conditions, a rapid review is not typically appropriate when a full literature review and synthesis is indicated (Ganann et al., 2010; Patnode et al., 2018).

Exemplar

The following rapid review of population surveys of indigenous populations in four countries assesses what information was collected to inform the development of mental health services. The reviewers determined that indicators of quality of care being provided for indigenous populations require more systematic collection.

- McIntyre, C., Harris, M. G., Baxter, A. J., Leske, S., Diminic, S., Gone, J. P., Hunter, E., & Whiteford, H. (2017). Assessing service use for mental health by indigenous populations in Australia, Canada, New Zealand and the United States of America: A rapid review of population surveys. *Health Research Policy and Systems, 15*(1), 67-017–0233-5. https://doi.org/10.1186/s12961-017-0233-5

  www.ncbi.nlm.nih.gov/pmc/articles/PMC5544983/pdf/12961_2017_Article_233.pdf

Realist Review

A realist review (also known as realist synthesis) is a theory-driven, iterative review that assesses programs, interventions, services, and policies (Jagosh, 2019). A realist review aims to enable evidence-informed healthcare and increase understanding of the causal mechanisms that impact complex interventions and strategies, exploring how interventions work and under what conditions (e.g., study settings and designs), as well as the outcomes of the interventions (Jagosh, 2019; Noble & Smith, 2018; Rycroft-Malone et al., 2012; Samnani et al., 2017). A realist review is designed to filter and synthesize evidence about complex contexts and the interrelated mechanisms of interventions that underlie implementation activities, and to identify the reasons that a complex intervention succeeds or fails in a certain setting. Findings can help to inform choices about use of interventions, as well as future research directions (Rycroft-Malone et al., 2012; Samnani et al., 2017). In a realist review, the search and appraisal of evidence is purposive and theoretically-driven. The search in a realist review should be extensive, including a range of relevant databases and hand searching, along with attempts to identify relevant unpublished literature (Noble & Smith, 2018). Multiple data sources and types of evidence can be included in a realist review (Rycroft-Malone et al., 2012).

Advantages

A realist review approach is rooted in both philosophy and social sciences; this provides a flexible, encompassing approach to be able to explain what will work (and what will likely not work) for specific groups of people across varied circumstances and settings. The emphasis is not on controlling for specific events, but rather providing a framework to understand the realities that specific persons and groups encounter in different situations (Rycroft-Malone et al., 2012), allowing for the new idea generation to address distinct healthcare concerns (Jagosh, 2019).

Challenges

A realist review can be complex and contextually specific. A realist review does not have tightly scripted instructions; this can be challenging, particularly for the novice reviewer. The process required to complete a quality realist review can be time consuming and requires multiple resources, including a multidisciplinary team. Each member of a realist review team brings distinct perspectives and needs to have the abilities to both understand and thoughtfully discuss program and intervention implementation, as well as explore a selected topic from a theoretical viewpoint (Jagosh, 2019).

Exemplar

The following realist review is focused on implementation theories, specifically, the factors that facilitate or hinder the implementation of advance care planning conversations among patients diagnosed with end-stage kidney disease. The reviewers conducted a theory synthesis to explain and provide support for the implementation of an intervention for advance care planning. The reviewers identify two stages of the intervention: (a) training for healthcare professionals, and (b) focus and goal of the approach used for implementation.

- O'Halloran, P., Noble, H., Norwood, K., Maxwell, P., Shields, J., Fogarty, D., Murtagh, F., Morton, R., & Brazil, K. (2018). Advance care planning with patients who have end-stage kidney disease: A systematic realist review. *Journal of Pain and Symptom Management*, 56(5), 795–807.e18. https://doi.org/10.1016/j.jpainsymman.2018 .07.008

   www.ncbi.nlm.nih.gov/pmc/articles/PMC6203056/?report=printable

Scoping Review

[Other names: Scoping Study]
A scoping review is designed to evaluate the landscape of literature available on a particular topic. A scoping review seeks to determine the extent and type of literature available and may also include locating in-progress research. Through providing a preliminary assessment of the potential size, scope, and identification of the characteristics of the available literature, a scoping review can determine a suitable and timely topic for a more structured review (Grant & Booth, 2009; Noble & Smith, 2018). The thoroughness or completeness of a scoping review is determined by both the time dedicated, and restraints or limitations placed on the scope of the review. Generally, a scoping review includes a comprehensive search strategy, intending to retrieve a wide breadth of literature, which may or may not include in-progress research; a scoping review does not, however, synthesize the included literature (Grant & Booth, 2009; Smith & Noble, 2016) and may not include a formal critical appraisal (Grant & Booth, 2009). A single reviewer may choose to screen titles/abstracts and full texts in comparison to a dual reviewer approach. While using only a single rather than dual approach can introduce an additional and is generally not considered a "gold standard" approach, it is an efficient strategy to reviewing the literature prior to conducting a more rigorous literature review. The scoping review approach is gaining increasing respect in international review arenas. Scoping reviews can be used to organize existing evidence before conducting a systematic review. The scoping review process allows a reviewer to confidently characterize the state of the science and determine an evidence gap, or question, to address via a more rigorous review type. A scoping review can be used to display and

describe different types of evidence such as emerging evidence, evidence designed to inform clinical decision-making and/or policy-making, and broad evidence overviews, with intent to identify and address gaps in the available evidence (Peters et al., 2020).

Advantages

A scoping review can aid in assessing the utility and achievability of completing a full systematic review on a given topic (Noble & Smith, 2018). A scoping review is also useful when time is limited and there is a need to have at least a preliminary understanding of the literature on a healthcare topic.

Challenges

While the emphasis of a scoping review is on providing a descriptive overview, depending on the restrictions placed by the reviewer, this type of review can be limited in the breadth and depth of literature captured. Therefore, important literature on a topic may be missed, especially if it is in a lesser-known database or the grey literature (Tricco et al., 2016). This factor may impact the accuracy of evidence gap identification and recommendations for future reviews.

Exemplar

The following scoping review exemplar assesses the breadth and depth of literature in an area of vaccine distribution. Specifically studied are the immunization systems supply chains in sub-Saharan Africa. Recommendations are based on findings for system redesign that not only improve the availability for vaccines but also reduce cost associated with vaccine distribution.

- Vouking, M. Z., Mengue, C. M. A., Yauba, S., Edengue, J. M., Dicko, M., Dicko, H. M., & Wiysonge, C. S. (2019). Interventions to increase the distribution of vaccines in sub-Saharan Africa: A scoping review. *The Pan African Medical Journal, 32,* 14. https://doi.org/10.11604/pamj.2019.32.14.17225

  www.ncbi.nlm.nih.gov/pmc/articles/PMC6522164/pdf/PAMJ-32-14.pdf

State-of-the-Art Review

A state-of-the-art review addresses only current and contemporary topics, with emphasis on recent literature. The state-of-the-art review exists in many ways in contrast with the historical review, which overviews a substantial timeline and development of a topic. Rather, a state-of-the-art review aims to convey the current state of the knowledge regarding a topic, with the intent to offer readers not only a summary of the recent state of the science, but also new perspectives on a contemporary and highly relevant issue. A state-of-the-art review sets forth priorities, and similar to mapping and scoping reviews, highlights areas requiring further primary research and rigorous reviews.

The state-of-the-art review includes a comprehensive search of current literature. A formal quality assessment can be present but is not required (Grant & Booth, 2009).

Advantages

A state-of-the-art review is valuable for those who are new to a subject area, as reviewers can quickly ascertain a sense of the volume of available literature and key findings on a topic from a single review article. A state-of-the-art review can be particularly useful for those who are seeking to identify potential opportunities for selecting questions and methods for currently relevant research topics (Grant & Booth, 2009).

Challenges

In a state-of-the-art review, the reviewer may choose to narrow the timeframe for the search method. If the reviewer searches and selects articles from one primary point in time or over a relatively short time period, it is possible that the review may not fully capture or can potentially distort the reader's understanding of the historical development of a topic, as important evidence may exist outside of the limited selected timeframe (Grant & Booth, 2009). Further, the number of data sources included may be limited and therefore can produce a diminished or incomplete perspective on the overall understanding of a selected topic or question.

Exemplar

In the following state-of-the-art review, the reviewers assessed literature from 2007 to 2017 to examine how eHealth has been leveraged for adults with hearing impairments who use hearing aids. The reviewers conceptually defined eHealth by using the World Health Organization (WHO) definition. The reviewers note that the growing interest in the area of eHealth in the setting of hearing impairment has resulted in an increasing number of publications throughout the decade reviewed (2007–2017). The reviewers report that further research regarding the efficacy of eHealth use in clinical practice with patients who use hearing aids is needed.

- Paglialonga, A., Cleveland Nielsen, A., Ingo, E., Barr, C., & Laplante-Levesque, A. (2018). eHealth and the hearing aid adult patient journey: A state-of-the-art review. *Biomedical Engineering Online, 17*(1), 101-018–0531-3. https://doi.org/10.1186/s12938-018-0531-3

  www.ncbi.nlm.nih.gov/pmc/articles/PMC6069792

Systematic Review

The systematic review is the most rigorous type of literature review. The systematic review uses only explicit and reproducible methodology and serves as the gold standard of literature reviews (Higgins & Green, 2011; Noble & Smith, 2018). The systematic review is predicated on using explicit criteria to systematically search all sources of evidence and critically appraise, summarize, and synthesize study findings to address a highly focused review purpose and question (Cronin et al., 2008; Noble & Smith, 2018). In a systematic review, the reviewer follows a rigorous protocol to comprehensively and exhaustively search the literature, attempting to identify all studies that meet eligibility criteria (Higgins & Green, 2011; Higgins et al., 2011). The systematic review can provide a comprehensive list of published and unpublished studies relating to a particular topic, purpose, or question (Cronin et al., 2008). The systematic review focuses primarily on experimental studies, such as randomized controlled trials (Souza et al., 2010), but may also include other study types (as discussed elsewhere in this text). A systematic review can include not only randomized controlled trials, but also non-randomized designs (case-control, interrupted time-series studies) and prospective before-and-after designs (Littell et al., 2008). Critical appraisal and quality assessment factor into the assessment of article eligibility, as a systematic review aims to include studies with only valid, reliable, and high-quality data. Many, but not all, systematic reviews contain a meta-analysis (Littell et al., 2008). The term "systematic" may be seen in the title of other types of literature reviews, implying that these literature reviews underwent a systematic process, though they may or may not meet all criteria of a "systematic review," per se.

Due to the scientific importance of systematic reviews, many comprehensive books have been written detailing precisely how to rigorously complete systematic reviews. Also, many global organizations provide extensive instruction on systematic review conduct, including but not limited to the Centre for Reviews and Dissemination, Cochrane Library, and the Joanna Briggs Institute. To expand and strengthen your understanding of systematic review principles and processes, you can consult the websites of these established organizations for supplemental information and guidance.

There are many different reasons that a systematic review may be undertaken. As noted in Boxes 2.1 to 2.3, systematic reviews can serve different purposes. Reasons include reviewing the efficacy and potential adverse effects of interventions, etiology and risk reviews, prognosis reviews, and diagnostic test accuracy reviews, among many others. Methodological evidence, prevalence and incidence, and public health interventions can be studied using systematic reviews. Other types of systematic reviews include economic analyses, text and opinion, and policy reviews. Importantly, a systematic review may include qualitative reviews and synthesize studies that employ different qualitative methodologies.

Advantages

In a systematic review, a large quantity of scientific information is gathered, evaluated, and synthesized into a shorter document. This document allows nurses, healthcare professionals, and health policy experts to stay abreast of new scientific developments without having to independently locate and synthesize often overwhelming amounts of literature (Bettany-Saltikov & McSherry, 2012; Bolderston, 2008). Further, because of the systematic nature and methodological transparency, bias can more easily be detected and therefore reduced (Littell et al., 2008). A systematic review allows for increased power and precision in estimating effects and risks (Bolderston, 2008).

Challenges

Even the most rigorously completed systematic review cannot compensate for sub-optimal quality of the included original studies (Littell et al., 2008). Combining results across varied study types, treatments, samples, settings, and outcomes may be complicated and typically requires training, or at minimum, working with skilled systematic reviewers. Lastly, a systematic review requires regular updates in order to reflect the current state of the knowledge on a given topic.

Exemplar

Multiple systematic review exemplars reside within the Centre for Reviews and Dissemination, Cochrane Library, and the Joanna Briggs Institute, as well as other reputable databases. Hand hygiene has been a part of the ongoing discussion of providing safe healthcare for centuries; as a topic of consistent relevance regarding infection control, multiple primary studies of varying quality have been conducted in diverse healthcare settings across the globe. Systematic reviews have been particularly useful in helping to cull, evaluate, and draw conclusions from this expansive evidence regarding hand hygiene across settings. Recently, Cochrane Library reviewers updated a systematic review on hand hygiene compliance.

- Gould, D. J., Moralejo, D., Drey, N., Chudleigh, J. H., & Taljaard, M. (2017). Interventions to improve hand hygiene compliance in patient care. *The Cochrane Database of Systematic Reviews, 9,* CD005186. https://doi.org/10.1002/14651858.CD005186.pub4

  www.ncbi.nlm.nih.gov/pmc/articles/PMC6483670/pdf/CD005186.pdf

Umbrella Review

[Other names: Overview of Reviews; Review of Reviews; Systematic Review Synthesis; Summary of Systematic Reviews]

An umbrella review is designed to compile, extract, appraise, compare, and synthesize into one document the evidence from multiple existing literature reviews. As a point of emphasis, the analytical units of an umbrella review are literature reviews, not primary research studies, as is commonly seen in other literature review and synthesis types and is generally aimed at informing readers on a specific clinical condition or topic (Aromataris et al., 2020; Biondi-Zoccai, 2016; Bougioukas et al., 2018). An umbrella review aims to create an overall picture of the published literature review findings regarding a particular topic, question, or phenomenon, comparing and contrasting findings of relevant literature reviews. An umbrella review assesses whether published literature reviews address similar review questions independently, observe similar results, and arrive at generally comparable conclusions. An umbrella review provides a ready means for healthcare stakeholders to form an understanding of a broad topic area, which facilitates and supports decision-making. An umbrella review, however, is not intended to repeat the searches, assessments, or conclusions drawn from included literature reviews (Aromataris et al., 2020). An umbrella review can include diverse literature review types (e.g., qualitative reviews, quantitative reviews). Importantly, the quality appraisal process within an umbrella review may entail evaluation of reviews included, as well as an evaluation of the individual primary studies that were included in the literature reviews (analytic units of the umbrella review) (Grant & Booth, 2009).

Advantages

An umbrella review can be useful in aggregating published reviews, particularly when a review purpose or question is very broad and many literature reviews have already been conducted on the topic area (Noble & Smith, 2018; Smith et al., 2011). An umbrella review can help expand identification of what is known versus unknown on a topic and can provide direction for future research and practice (Grant & Booth, 2009).

Challenges

Discrepancies in eligibility criteria across included literature reviews can complicate analysis and interpretation in an umbrella review (Noble & Smith, 2018). Similar to systematic reviews that are limited by the quality of data included, an umbrella review is limited by the breadth and systematicity of the search, as well as the rigor of the included reviews (Conn & Coon Sells, 2014b). Reviewers are advised to carefully document overlap in primary studies included in the literature reviews that are included in the umbrella review (Conn & Coon Sells, 2014b). This documentation is intended primarily to avoid duplicity leading to the inflated appearance that more primary studies exist on a topic or question than in actuality are available. In other words, if 15 reviews are included in an umbrella review, while the total number of primary studies included in all 15 reviews may be 100, 20 of those studies may have appeared more than once. The reviewer should explicitly document the total number of primary studies, without double counting (Conn & Coon Sells, 2014b).

Exemplar

The following umbrella review assesses the effectiveness of psychological interventions for pain reduction. This umbrella review includes a total of 38 papers which contributed 150 meta-analyses and resulted in 865 individual study estimates. Given the high number of literature reviews completed on this topic, an umbrella review was selected to evaluate and synthesize the findings of the already existing literature reviews.

- Markozannes, G., Aretouli, E., Rintou, E., Dragioti, E., Damigos, D., Ntzani, E., Evangelou, E., Tsilidis, K. K. (2017). An umbrella review of the literature on the effectiveness of psychological interventions for pain reduction. *BMC Psychology, 5*(1), 31-017–0200-5. https://doi.org/10.1186/s40359-017-0200-5

  bmcpsychology.biomedcentral.com/track/pdf/10.1186/s40359-017-0200-5

Selecting a Type of Literature Review and Synthesis

Given the myriad of literature review type options, it may initially be overwhelming to determine which type you will select. There are several important factors to consider

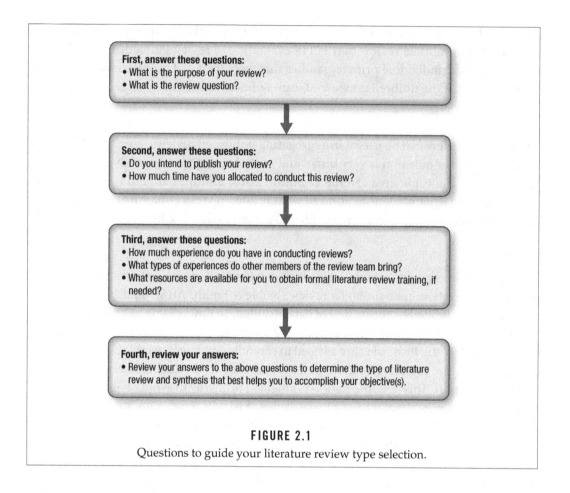

FIGURE 2.1

Questions to guide your literature review type selection.

when making your literature review type decision. Like all pursuits, with knowledge and exposure, this decision will be made more understandable and manageable. To begin, it may be useful for you to answer some questions specific to your purposes (Figure 2.1).

In order to proceed in knowing which literature review type to use, it is first essential to have already established a clear review purpose and question. Considerable discussion with your review team members is required to achieve consensus around an appropriate review question. It is also useful to think about the motivation driving your review question. Are you trying to determine the next step in your research? Are you trying to obtain information to guide an evidence-based clinical decision? Do you need to rapidly provide information to advise a policy decision? Are you writing a comprehensive background for a research project? Establishing a clear rationale for the review will help you to determine which type of literature review to conduct. If you intend to publish your literature review, it is advisable to carefully prepare a protocol prior to commencing the literature review and synthesis process. Also remember to follow the author instructions and style guide for target journals, referencing the standards of acceptable reviews for publication.

RESOURCES

Resources such as financial support and available time for you and other review team members, play a notable role in determining what type of literature review to conduct. Resource availability or lack thereof will limit or expand your possibilities for conducting certain types of resource-intensive literature reviews. The amount of prior experience you and your review team have in completing literature reviews and syntheses will also inform what type of literature review and synthesis you might lean toward. If you determine that you need to conduct a systematic review, it will be beneficial to locate the resources needed to obtain formal systematic review training or include review teams members with this training and experience.

By answering these questions, you will have completed the initial considerations necessary to determine the optimal literature review type and the best fit to the resources available to you and your review team. After considering and answering these questions, if you remain uncertain as to which type of review you should select, you might seek out additional expertise from those with literature review experience to provide guidance in determining the best literature review type for your review purpose and question.

ACTIVITIES
Activity I

You are a healthcare professional that has been tasked by your organization's administration to better understand patient safety culture. As you start your initial scan of the literature, you quickly locate the following two literature reviews recently published on the topic of patient safety culture. The first publication is a systematic review and meta-analysis addressing how healthcare professionals perceive patient safety, as measured by a Hospital Survey on Patient Safety Culture. The second publication is a scoping review exploring patient safety culture, focusing on older people in care homes.

- Okuyama, J. H. H., Galvao, T. F., & Silva, M. T. (2018). Healthcare professionals' perception of patient safety measured by the hospital survey on patient safety culture: A systematic review and meta-analysis. *The Scientific World Journal, 2018,* 9156301. https://doi.org/10.1155/2018/9156301

  www.ncbi.nlm.nih.gov/pmc/articles/PMC6076892/pdf/TSWJ2018-9156301.pdf

- Gartshore, E., Waring, J., & Timmons, S. (2017). Patient safety culture in care homes for older people: A scoping review. *BMC Health Services Research, 17*(1), 752-017-2713-2. https://doi.org/10.1186/s12913-017-2713-2

  www.bmchealthservres.biomedcentral.com/track/pdf/10.1186/s12913-017-2713-2.pdf

Before you proceed with your project, you decide to read and compare these reviews. As you do so, think about the following questions. If possible, also discuss these questions in a group of peers and/or colleagues.

1. What question is addressed in each review?
2. Do you think that the reviewers used the correct literature review type to address their review question? Why or why not?
3. What are the advantages and disadvantages of each of these types of literature review (i.e., systematic, scoping)?
4. What are the main differences between these two reviews? What similarities do you note?
5. What have you learned from these reviews that will guide your next steps in your organizational task?
6. Was there a synthesis in either or both literature reviews?

Activity II

You are preparing to conduct a literature review and synthesis as part of your academic program requirements. As you consider the type of literature review that you might conduct, consider the following questions. If possible, also discuss these questions with peers and/or colleagues.

1. What is your motivation for conducting this particular literature review, within the context of this assignment? Why this particular review purpose and/or question?
2. What are you hoping to accomplish with this literature review and synthesis?
3. What are two or three possible literature review types that you might select? What might be beneficial in selecting each particular literature review type, in contrast to others?

SUMMARY POINTS

A multitude of literature review and synthesis types are available for you to explore and pursue. The information provided in this chapter is a cursory overview and introduction to different types of literature reviews, providing a brief overview of each of the most widely used types of literature reviews in nursing and other healthcare professional and policy arenas. Systematic reviews are recognized as the gold standard for literature reviews, due to their methodological rigor and reproducibility. Different types of literature reviews described in this chapter may also follow a systematic process. We hope that this provides you with a point of reference in choosing the type of literature review you plan to conduct and hopefully publish.

- There is a multitude of different types of literature reviews and syntheses. Different types of literature reviews and syntheses have a collection of unique features.

- The various types of literature reviews and syntheses share commonalities. All literature reviews require the identification of a central topic, review purpose, and question. Also, a justification should be provided for conducting the literature review and synthesis. Each review involves determination of inclusion, review and appraisal of the literature, data extraction and synthesis. The process and level of depth required of each of these steps can vary among different types of reviews.

- Consider when a literature review and synthesis is needed. To determine this need, you might begin by evaluating the number (and quality) of existing primary studies and literature reviews that could contribute to your own literature review and synthesis.

- In this chapter, an overview of the features, advantages, and challenges of 14 different literature review types are described, along with an exemplar. Leading global organizations provide detailed instructions for conducting literature reviews and syntheses. Using a systematic review process is considered the gold standard when undertaking a literature review and synthesis.

- Determining which type of literature review and synthesis to conduct can be challenging. Questions are provided to guide the reviewer toward determining the optimal type of literature review and synthesis for your particular motivation, review purpose, and question.

REFERENCES

Aromataris, E., Fernandez, R., Godfrey, C., Holly, C., Khalil, H., & Tungpunkom, P. (2020). Chapter 10: Umbrella reviews. In E. Aromataris, & Z. Munn (Eds.), *JBI manual for evidence synthesis*. JBI. https://synthesismanual.jbi.global. https://doi.org/10.46658/JBIMES-20-11

Aromataris, E., & Munn, Z. (2020a). Chapter 1: JBI systematic reviews. In E. Aromataris, & Z. Munn (Eds.), *JBI manual for evidence synthesis*. JBI. https://synthesismanual.jbi.global. https://doi.org/10.46658/JBIMES -20-02

Aromataris, E., & Munn, Z. (Eds.). (2020b). *JBI manual for evidence synthesis*. JBI. https://synthesismanual.jbi. global. https://doi.org/10.46658/JBIMES-20-01

Aveyard, H., & Bradbury-Jones, C. (2019). An analysis of current practices in undertaking literature reviews in nursing: Findings from a focused mapping review and synthesis. *BMC Medical Research Methodology*, *19*(1), 105-019-0751-7. https://doi.org/10.1186/s12874-019-0751-7

Barnett-Page, E., & Thomas, J. (2009). Methods for the synthesis of qualitative research: A critical review. *BMC Medical Research Methodology*, *9*, 59-2288-9-59. https://doi.org/10.1186/1471-2288-9-59

Bettany-Saltikov, J., & McSherry, R. (2012). *How to do a systematic literature review in nursing: A step-by-step guide*. Open University Press.

Biondi-Zoccai, G. (Ed.). (2016). *Umbrella reviews: Evidence synthesis with overviews of reviews and meta-epidemiologic studies*. Springer.

Boland, A., Cherry, M. G., & Dickson, R. (2017). *Doing a systematic review: A student's guide* (2nd ed.). Sage.

Bolderston, A. (2008). Writing an effective literature review. *Journal of Medical Imaging and Radiation Sciences*, *39*(2), 86–92. https://doi.org/S1939-8654(08)00057-X

Bougioukas, K. I., Liakos, A., Tsapas, A., Ntzani, E., & Haidich, A. B. (2018). Preferred reporting items for overviews of systematic reviews including harms checklist: A pilot tool to be used for balanced reporting of benefits and harms. *Journal of Clinical Epidemiology*, *93*, 9–24. https://doi.org/S0895-4356(17)30798-9

Centre for Reviews and Dissemination, University of York. (2009). *Systematic reviews: CRD's guidance for undertaking reviews in health care*. CRD University of York.

Cochrane Library. (2021). *About cochrane reviews*. https://www.cochranelibrary.com/about/about-cochrane-reviews

Conn, V. S., & Coon Sells, T. G. (2014a). Is it time to write a review article? *Western Journal of Nursing Research*, *36*(4), 435–439. https://doi.org/10.1177/0193945913519060

Conn, V. S., & Coon Sells, T. G. (2014b). WJNR welcomes umbrella reviews. *Western Journal of Nursing Research*, *36*(2), 147–151. https://doi.org/10.1177/0193945913506968

Cronin, P., Ryan, F., & Coughlan, M. (2008). Undertaking a literature review: A step-by-step approach. *British Journal of Nursing (Mark Allen Publishing)*, *17*(1), 38–43. https://doi.org/10.12968/bjon.2008.17.1.28059

Doyle, L., Brady, A., & Byrne, G. (2016). An overview of mixed methods research - revisited. *Journal of Research in Nursing*, *21*(8), 623–635. https://doi.org/10.1177/1744987116667425

Ferrari, R. (2015). Writing narrative style literature reviews. *Medical Writing*, *24*(4), 230–235. https://doi.org/10.1179/2047480615Z.000000000329

Ganann, R., Ciliska, D., & Thomas, H. (2010). Expediting systematic reviews: Methods and implications of rapid reviews. *Implementation Science*, *5*, 56-5908-5-56. https://doi.org/10.1186/1748-5908-5-56

Grant, M. J., & Booth, A. (2009). A typology of reviews: An analysis of 14 review types and associated methodologies. *Health Information and Libraries Journal*, *26*(2), 91–108. https://doi.org/10.1111/j.1471-1842.2009.00848.x

Hailey, D., Corabian, P., Harstall, C., & Schneider, W. (2000). The use and impact of rapid health technology assessments. *International Journal of Technology Assessment in Health Care*, *16*(2), 651–656. https://doi.org/10.1017/s0266462300101205

Hart, C. (2018). *Doing a literature review: Releasing the research imagination* (2nd ed.). Sage.

Higgins, J. P. T., & Green, S. (2011). *Cochrane handbook for systematic reviews of interventions Version 5.1.0.* www.cochrane-handbook.org/

Higgins, J. P. T., Green, S., & Green, S. (2011). *Cochrane handbook for systematic review of interventions Version 5.1.0.* http://handbook.cochrane.org/

Jagosh, J. (2019). Realist synthesis for public health: Building an ontologically deep understanding of how programs work, for whom, and in which contexts. *Annual Review of Public Health*, *40*, 361–372. https://doi.org/10.1146/annurev-publhealth-031816-044451

Jesson, J., & Lacey, F. (2006). How to do (or not to do) a critical literature review. *Pharmacy Education*, *6*(2), 139–148.

Littell, J. H., Corcoran, J., & Pillai, V. (2008). *Systematic reviews and meta-analysis.* Oxford University Press.

Lockwood, C., Porrit, K., Munn, Z., Rittenmeyer, L., Salmond, S., Bjerrum, M., Loveday, H., Carrier, J., & Stannard, D. (2020). Chapter 2: Systematic reviews of qualitative evidence. In E. Aromataris, & Z. Munn (Eds.), *JBI manual for evidence synthesis.* JBI. https://synthesismanual.jbi.global. https://doi.org/10.46658/JBIMES-20-03

Moher, D., Shamseer, L., Clarke, M., Ghersi, D., Liberati, A., Petticrew, M., Shekelle, P., Steward, L. A., & PRISMA-P Group. (2015). Preferred reporting items for systematic review and meta-analysis protocols (PRISMA-P) 2015 statement. *Systematic Reviews*, *4*, 1-4053-4-1. https://doi.org/10.1186/2046-4053-4-1

Noble, H., & Smith, J. (2018). Reviewing the literature: Choosing a review design. *Evidence-Based Nursing*, *21*(2), 39–41. https://doi.org/10.1136/eb-2018-102895

Noblitt, G. W., & Hare, R. D. (1988). *Meta-ethnography: Synthesizing qualitative studies.* Sage.

Patnode, C. D., Eder, M. L., Walsh, E. S., Viswanathan, M., & Lin, J. S. (2018). The use of rapid review methods for the U.S. preventive services task force. *American Journal of Preventive Medicine*, *54*(1S1), S19–S25. https://doi.org/10.1016/j.amepre.2017.07.024

Pautasso, M. (2013). Ten simple rules for writing a literature review. *PLoS Computational Biology*, *9*(7), e1003149. https://doi.org/10.1371/journal.pcbi.1003149

Pearson, A., White, H., Bath-Hextall, F., Salmond, S., Apostolo, J., & Kirkpatrick, P. (2015). A mixed-methods approach to systematic reviews. *International Journal of Evidence-Based Healthcare*, *13*(3), 121–131. https://doi.org/10.1097/XEB.0000000000000052

Peters, M. D. J., Godfrey, C., McInerney, P., Munn, Z., Tricco, A. C., & Khalil, H. (2020). Chapter 11: Scoping reviews. In E. Aromataris & Z. Munn (Eds.), *JBI manual for evidence synthesis.* JBI. https://synthesismanual.jbi.global. https://doi.org/10.46658/JBIMES-20-12

Royle, P., & Waugh, N. (2003). Literature searching for clinical and cost-effectiveness studies used in health technology assessment reports carried out for the National Institute for Clinical Excellence appraisal system. *Health Technology Assessment (Winchester, England)*, *7*(34), 1–51. https://doi.org/10.3310/hta7340

Russell, C. L. (2005). An overview of the integrative research review. *Progress in Transplantation (Aliso Viejo, Calif.), 15*(1), 8–13.

Rycroft-Malone, J., McCormack, B., Hutchinson, A. M., DeCorby, K., Bucknall, T. K., Kent, B., Schultz, A., Snelgroe-Clarke, E., Stetler, C. B., Titler, M., Wallin, L., & Wilson, V. (2012). Realist synthesis: Illustrating the method for implementation research. *Implementation Science, 7,* 33-5908-7-33. https://doi.org/10.1186/1748-5908-7-33

Samnani, S. S., Vaska, M., Ahmed, S., & Turin, T. C. (2017). Review typology: The basic types of reviews for synthesizing evidence for the purpose of knowledge translation. *Journal of the College of Physicians and Surgeons--Pakistan, 27*(10), 635–641.

Sandelowski, M. (2014). Unmixing mixed-methods research. *Research in Nursing & Health, 37*(1), 3–8. https://doi.org/10.1002/nur.21570

Sandelowski, M., Voils, C. I., & Barroso, J. (2006). Defining and designing mixed research synthesis. *Research in the Schools: A Nationally Refereed Journal Sponsored by the Mid-South Educational Research Association and the University of Alabama, 13*(1), 29.

Saunders, M. N. K., & Rojon, C. (2011). On the attributes of a critical literature review. *Coaching: An International Journal of Theory, Research and Practice, 4*(2), 156–162. https://doi.org/10.1080/17521882.2011.596485

Smith, J., & Noble, H. (2016). Reviewing the literature. *Evidence-Based Nursing, 19*(1), 2–3. https://doi.org/10.1136/eb-2015-102252

Smith, V., Devane, D., Begley, C. M., & Clarke, M. (2011). Methodology in conducting a systematic review of systematic reviews of healthcare interventions. *BMC Medical Research Methodology, 11*(1), 15-2288-11-15. https://doi.org/10.1186/1471-2288-11-15

Souza, M. T., Silva, M. D., & Carvalho, R. (2010). Integrative review: What is it? How to do it? *Einstein (Sao Paulo, Brazil), 8*(1), 102–106. https://doi.org/10.1590/S1679-45082010RW1134

Topfer, L. A., Parada, A., Menon, D., Noorani, H., Perras, C., & Serra-Prat, M. (1999). Comparison of literature searches on quality and costs for health technology assessment using the MEDLINE and EMBASE databases. *International Journal of Technology Assessment in Health Care, 15*(2), 297–303.

Torraco, R. J. (2016). Writing integrative literature reviews: Using the past and present to explore the future. *Integrative Literature Review, 15*(4), 404–428. https://doi.org/10.1177/1534484316671606

Tricco, A. C., Langlois, E. V., & Straus, S. E. (Eds.). (2017). *Rapid reviews to strengthen health policy and systems: A practical guide.* World Health Organization Licence: CC BY-NC-SA 3.0 IGO. http://apps.who.int/iris/bitstream/handle/10665/258698/9789241512763-eng.pdf?sequence=1

Tricco, A. C., Soobiah, C., Antony, J., Cogo, E., MacDonald, H., Lillie, E., Tran, J., D'Souza, J., Hui, W., Perrier, L., Welch, V., Horsley, T., Straus, S. E., & Kastner, M. (2016). A scoping review identifies multiple emerging knowledge synthesis methods, but few studies operationalize the method. *Journal of Clinical Epidemiology, 73,* 19–28. https://doi.org/10.1016/j.jclinepi.2015.08.030

Watt, A., Cameron, A., Sturm, L., Lathlean, T., Babidge, W., Blamey, S., Facey, K., Hailey, D., Norderhaug, I., & Maddern, G. (2008). Rapid reviews versus full systematic reviews: An inventory of current methods and practice in health technology assessment. *International Journal of Technology Assessment in Health Care, 24*(2), 133–139. https://doi.org/10.1017/S0266462308080185

Whittemore, R. (2005). Combining evidence in nursing research: Methods and implications. *Nursing Research, 54*(1), 56–62. https://doi.org/00006199-200501000-00008

Whittemore, R., & Knafl, K. (2005). The integrative review: Updated methodology. *Journal of Advanced Nursing, 52*(5), 546–553. https://doi.org/10.1111/j.1365-2648.2005.03621.x

Wong, G., Greenhalgh, T., Westhorp, G., Buckingham, J., & Pawson, R. (2013). RAMESES publication standards: Meta-narrative reviews. *BMC Medicine, 11,* 20-7015-11-20. https://doi.org/10.1186/1741-7015-11-20

3

Preparing for the Literature Review and Synthesis

Susan W. Buchholz and Kirsten A. Dickins

Part of making the commitment to writing a literature review and synthesis is understanding the "why" that is driving your participation, which is arguably among your most important preliminary decisions.

CHAPTER OUTLINE

This chapter provides step-by-step guidance on completing the first stages of your literature review and synthesis. When first making the commitment, it is advisable to assess the time, skills, environmental resources, and financial support necessary to successfully complete your literature review and synthesis. Understanding your "why" for conducting the literature review will guide you in selecting the topic area. An initial informal literature search will assist in defining the review purpose and formulation of the review question. You will learn to select which type of literature review and synthesis is most suited to your review purpose and question, and to consider opportunities for both novel reviews and updating prior original reviews. Lastly, you will gain an understanding of how to form an optimized review team, as well as how to prepare a review protocol that provides detailed guidance for the conduct of your literature review.

LEARNING OBJECTIVES

In this chapter, we lay out the steps required to prepare for completing a literature review and synthesis. By the end of this chapter, you will be able to:

- Understand why it is critical to begin by making the commitment to completing your literature review and synthesis

- Assess which resources will be necessary to successfully complete your literature review and synthesis

- Describe how to select an appropriate topic area

- Execute successfully an initial informal literature search

- Discuss how to define the purpose for a literature review and synthesis

- Appreciate the steps necessary to formulating and finalizing the review question

- Recognize how to determine what type of literature review and synthesis is best suited to your review purpose and question

- Identify when the completion of a novel review versus an original review update is indicated

- Comprehend how to prepare and follow a detailed review protocol

- Explain the importance of having a diverse review team with varied areas of expertise

MAKING THE COMMITMENT

Prior to beginning your literature review and synthesis, it is important to first fully appraise and understand the time and energy commitment that will be required; a substantial investment of these finite resources is required in order to comprehensively read and understand the literature on a given topic. While it can be the experts in a field who seem best poised to assume the task of completing a literature review, it is often rather the *expert-in-training* who benefits and grows most from undertaking this process, as they develop their area of expertise while contributing meaningfully to the state of the science (Pautasso, 2013). Ensuring that you have the time available to complete the review will increase the likelihood of successful completion. It may be useful prior to undertaking a review to complete a time inventory of your professional and personal

TABLE 3.1 TIME INVENTORY

Timeline	Current and future projects/commitments
Month 1	
Month 2	
Month 3	
Month 4	
Month 5	
Month 6	
Month 7	
Month 8	
Month 9	
Month 10	
Month 11	
Month 12	

commitments over the next year. In Table 3.1, you can complete a time inventory, considering and listing pre-existing commitments, projects that are currently underway, and likely future projects, in order to gain a sense of the feasibility of completing a review in the next year.

Part of making the commitment to writing a literature review and synthesis is understanding the "why" that is driving your participation, which is arguably among your most important preliminary decisions. The "why" that motivates your conducting a literature review and synthesis will have a noteworthy impact on the approach that you will take (Bolderston, 2008). For instance, whether you are preparing to complete your master's thesis or doctoral dissertation, intending to publish a research paper, develop clinical guidelines (Bolderston, 2008), or answer your own nursing or other question(s), may impact your review decisions. The "why" driving your review will influence the way in which you approach your initial steps, the resources that may be available to you, the extent of your review team expertise, and your anticipated dissemination process and venues. With a balanced assessment of the time and energy requirements, projected scientific contribution, professional growth opportunities, and personal motivations and goals, you will be able to reasonably determine whether it is appropriate timing for you to make the commitment to completing a literature review and synthesis. There are several potential reasons—or motivating "whys"— for conducting a literature review and synthesis, which each depend on what the reviewer intends to accomplish. Box 3.1 provides an overview of common reasons for conducting a literature review and synthesis (Booth et al., 2016; Hart, 2018).

BOX 3.1   REASONS FOR CONDUCTING A LITERATURE REVIEW AND SYNTHESIS

- Assess the breadth and depth of empirical literature.
- Develop a critical understanding of the literature relevant to one's research and/or clinical practice.
- Identify gaps in the literature that require further investigation.
- Ascertain the key variables of importance for further evaluation.
- Distinguish the methodologies used to explore a particular topic.
- Connect theoretical literature with a research question or clinical issue.
- Evaluate existing instruments that have been used to study a certain topic or question.
- Explore the relative contributions of individual publications within the context of the overall body of relevant literature.
- Attempt to mediate inconsistent findings apparent in the literature on a given topic or question.
- Provide a timeline or historical context for existing and projected future research.
- Develop and/or update evidence-based clinical guidelines.
- Support quality improvement efforts.
- Guide healthcare or public health policy decisions.

ASSESSING THE RESOURCES

As you thoroughly consider your commitment from all angles, we recommend that you carefully assess the resources that will be required to successfully complete your literature review and synthesis. Resources that are needed to conduct a literature review and synthesis include having the available time, skill set, or opportunity to develop or update prior skill sets; and reviewing team expertise and the environmental infrastructure; and ensuring financial support. As you consider each of these resources, document if each one present or not in your current context; if not, develop a plan to obtain the necessary resource(s), or how you will work around this resource limitation (Table 3.2)

Chief among these resource considerations is the *time commitment*—undoubtedly one of the most valuable and limited resources required to be successful in completing your literature review and synthesis. Earlier in this chapter, you completed a time inventory of professional and personal commitments over the next year; through this, you may have recognized just how limited your time is. At the outset of conducting a literature review, it may appear to be overwhelming for anyone: a student who has many competing demands ranging from course work, clinical training, and examinations, or a faculty member who is likely immersed in many other simultaneous research projects, teaching responsibilities, and mentoring roles. Time is a constant for all of us; we each have the same amount of time in every hour, day, week, month, and year. However, we each have unique and competing demands for our time, both professional and personal. Because of the degree of cognitive concentration required by a review, it may be important for you to schedule consistent time

TABLE 3.2 RESOURCES NECESSARY FOR CONDUCTING A LITERATURE REVIEW AND SYNTHESIS

Resources	Do you have these resources? If not, write a plan for how you will realistically obtain the resources, or how you will address resource limitations.
1. Time	
2. Skills	
3. Team	
4. Environment	
5. Finance	

during a set day or protect time on your calendar when you know yourself to be most productive. Like all large worthwhile projects, the literature review and synthesis process can be broken down into sequential manageable stages; taking this stepwise approach to your review may be beneficial (Boland et al., 2017; Booth et al., 2016). Committing to a set regular time(s) and allocating a consistent amount of time during this time block to work on the review will increase your likelihood of completing a thoughtful, quality literature review and synthesis. If needed, constructing a timeline of how you will complete the review over the course of a set amount of time (e.g., one year) may be helpful in realistically balancing the work required to complete your review along with your other professional and personal responsibilities. It is important to adhere to your proposed timeline to the greatest extent possible, as reviews can quickly become outdated with the rapid publication of related primary and secondary literature. In the case of a literature review that has become outdated with the passage of time, the review team may be in the difficult position of either trying to publish a review that is already considered outdated, or of having to return to the literature search stages in order to systematically identify and appraise recently published science—which can be time consuming.

The next consideration is regarding that of your skill level. If you are new to conducting literature reviews and syntheses, there are many opportunities available to improve your knowledge and skills in this domain. You may gain knowledge by reading a book such as this, or by perusing other books that are focused on a specific review type. There are also opportunities for knowledge and skill development available electronically, including enrolling in free or low-cost online courses, watching educational videos informed by literature review experts, or attending formal in-person literature review workshops and courses. If possible, it may be beneficial to identify a mentor, colleague, or peer who has experience in conducting literature reviews and syntheses, learning directly from this person's example and guidance on approach and style. If you have already developed and refined the skills necessary to successfully complete a quality literature review and synthesis, then quickly self-assess whether you will need to refresh or enhance those skills prior to beginning your literature review and synthesis. See Table 3.3 for a skills inventory and check-off, informed by Benner's Novice to Expert rankings (Benner, 2001). This table will help you to determine the domains in which you

TABLE 3.3 SKILL SET INVENTORY

	Novice	Advanced Beginner	Competent	Proficient	Expert
Defining the purpose					
Question formulation					
Search strategy development					
Search execution					
Information technology use					
Working with a review team					
Literature screening (title/abstract, full-text)					
Critical appraisal/quality assessment					
Data extraction					
Literature synthesis					
Manuscript preparation					
Determining dissemination venues					
Publication process (submission, revisions)					

are proficient and the areas in which you may benefit from continuing to build the skills needed for completion of a high quality literature review and synthesis.

After you have personally reflected on your time available and your skill level, we recommend that you turn your attention outward—toward leveraging the expertise around you and creating and maintaining an optimized review team. Your review team is critical to the successful completion of a high-quality literature review and synthesis. Later in this chapter we address the elements of composing a team that will enhance the strength of the review. Each team member needs to scan their scholastic domain and assess who is able to contribute to the review team at which level in each domain. Equally important, each team member must be willing and able to commit to sustaining engagement with the team until literature review and synthesis process completion.

In your next assessment of external supports, determining the level of environmental support is vital in ensuring the organizational resources available for the successful completion of your literature review. Environmental support includes access to relevant information technology including high-speed internet connectivity, screening and data extraction software, reference management software, electronic database access, and consultation opportunity if needed, such as with a medical librarian, statistician, and/or writing editors, as well as, potentially, a research assistant. If you are conducting your literature review under an existing systematic review organization, then you will likely have sufficient tools to be able to complete your review, as well as experts in the field who are able to answer your questions and guide you through the complexities of conducting a review. If you are in a university, hospital, or other organizational setting where resources are available for conducting reviews, then it is also likely that you will have sufficient environmental support. If you are in a setting in which resources are not as abundant or readily available, then it may be useful to strategize with faculty or administrators on how to address environmental support limitations. When needed, establishing contractual agreements regarding expectations for environmental support in exchange for set deliverables, such as the quality completion of your literature review and synthesis, may be advantageous.

Lastly, evaluating the potential for financial support may be useful, as funding for literature reviews and syntheses can be quite variable. If you are an experienced reviewer, then you may have the option of applying for federal or foundation grants that will support the completion of rigorous literature reviews and syntheses. For less experienced reviewers, there are still several necessary financial considerations. If you will require formal training, financial support is helpful for covering fees associated with online or in-person literature review courses or workshops. For faculty, you may be able to negotiate with your leadership/administration to cover a percentage of your effort to afford you more scholarship time to dedicate to your literature review. If other resources are not available within your environment, you may need to negotiate for costs associated with information technology access, consultation fees, and/or a research assistant(s). Other costs to consider are those related to dissemination of your literature review and synthesis, including attendance and presentations at conferences and fees associated with publication.

SELECTING THE TOPIC AREA

With a strong commitment in-place and a comprehensive understanding of the resources that are available to you, it is now time to identify the general topic area in which a literature review would meaningfully add to the science. A successfully completed literature review requires careful organization and planning from the outset, following well-defined steps beginning with identification of the topic area (Boland et al., 2017). It is often the case that reviewers are uncertain of how to start, specifically how to select a topic area (Cronin et al., 2008). The initial steps that you take toward your literature review and synthesis will be unique to your topic(s) of interest and areas of expertise; in most situations, you are generally free to choose a topic that interests you (Bolderston, 2008). The topic area may be informed by your clinical area of expertise, timely healthcare or health policy issue that you desire to better understand, or perhaps related to a pressing question that remains unanswered for you. Selecting your general topic area will inform each subsequent review stage, from determining the review purpose to crafting the review question, making it vital to firmly establish the topic area before proceeding to your next steps (Figure 3.1). It is worth noting that there is a lack of consensus regarding the precise order in which a review should be approached, such as whether you will determine your topic area prior to or after completing your initial informal literature search (Bolderston, 2008). We recommend that you begin with selecting a broad topic area that suits and

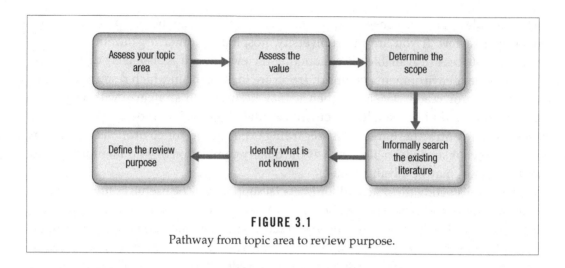

FIGURE 3.1

Pathway from topic area to review purpose.

BOX 3.2   COMPONENTS OF A LITERATURE REVIEW PROTOCOL

- Review title
- Review team members
- Background
- Purpose/aims +/- question
- Eligibility criteria
- Search strategy
- Data review/literature screening plan
- Data extraction tools/plan
- Critical appraisal/quality assessment tools/plan
- Data analysis/synthesis plan
- Literature language/country of origin
- Conflicts of interest
- Acknowledgments
- Current stage of the review

---

leverages both your interests and expertise, and then narrow your topic focus after the completion of an initial informal scan of the literature; these steps should happen prior to beginning to define your review purpose and question formulation. A framework may inform your review; for example, the use of the Logic Model by a doctor of nursing practice student, who is using the model to determine how to address a clinical question (Littell et al., 2008). Box 3.2 provides step-by-step early literature review instructions, from assessing your topic area to defining the review purpose and question.

Determining the relative value of a topic is imperative when selecting your topic, and it is necessary to seek out the input of expert leaders in your topic area (Higgins et al., 2019) to ensure consensus around the value of the topic, prior to refining your review purpose and question. Asking questions and seeking detailed information broadly from professionals with expertise in your topic area is worthwhile, as differing perspectives on the same topic can help to define a review purpose and question of value to the field. It is also beneficial to seek out opinions of interdisciplinary team members, who may offer insight from a different angle or approach to a review purpose and question within your selected topic area. If your topic area is highly related to a specific population, it may also add value to discuss the topic with members of this population group to begin thinking through the most pertinent and timely questions. As clinicians are trained to consider and integrate the input of patients (shared decision-making) in personalizing care plans, researchers are now more heavily emphasizing the input of members of certain populations or persons who will be potentially impacted by the outcomes and implementation of the review findings into practice.

Justifying the relevance of the review will necessarily involve focusing or limiting the scope of your literature review and selecting a perspective (Machi & McEnvoy, 2016). Determining the scope of your review requires considerable thought, as you want to establish parameters that are neither too general nor too specific. If the topic is too general, it may require an unreasonable amount of resources to address the review purpose and question within a realistic time period. Additionally, if a question is too broad, it may prove difficult to meaningfully synthesize all relevant, eligible literature. Conversely, it is equally important to not overly narrow the scope of a review, such that the yield of relevant literature is too small to thoughtfully synthesize. Throughout the process of selecting a topic, it is imperative to include only what is within the determined scope of your topic area, not that which is simply peripherally related or only indirectly related to your selected topic and the parameters of your review. As you move forward in selecting and refining your topic of interest, remember, it should be: (a) *interesting to you*—this topic must hold your attention over an extended period; (b) *valuable within your current or intended field of expertise*—beyond simple personal interest, the topic should hold value for stakeholders; (c) *well-defined*—if your topic is too broad or too narrow, and your database of articles too large or too small, it may ultimately reduce the relevance of your review; and (d) allow for generation of an *addressable review purpose and answerable question* concerning an existing problem or issue in your field.

CONDUCTING AN INITIAL INFORMAL LITERATURE SEARCH

Once you have selected your topic area, you will next work toward defining the purpose and question driving your literature review. As you have taken your time to select the topic area, you are likely entering this phase with a general understanding of the gaps in the literature. Still, we recommend that you take the time to complete an initial informal search of the literature. Through this initial informal literature search, you will ideally encounter recent seminal papers in your field that may call for a review as a next research step, or garner attention toward a particular dearth of empirical knowledge. As mentioned earlier, some reviewers may at this point complete a preliminary, unsystematic search of the literature prior to establishing the purpose. Others may have predetermined the purpose of their review, informed by a known gap within their research or clinical areas of expertise, or may be aware enough of the needs based upon their broad understanding of a given topic area. With either approach, it is imperative for the reviewer to understand where and how their review fits within the larger context of existing literature on the topic.

Informally Searching the Literature

Next, you will conduct a preliminary, relatively superficial search of the relevant literature (Bolderston, 2008). It is important to know that the existing research evidence to date is relevant to the general topic area on which you are focusing (Cooper, 2017). This search is intended to be a fairly limited review of the existing literature geared toward allowing you to locate, sift, sort, and read the literature, gleaning an understanding of the current state of the science. This process can be likened to performing a scoping search (Boland et al., 2017); while this initial search does not necessarily need to be systematic, a structured search method is preferred to ensure that you are locating the most relevant articles. Throughout this process, we recommend that you identify and catalogue the gold standard articles and additional articles that you find *most* relevant for your review; you will use these later as you develop and conduct a more formal, systematic search.

While your initial search is not intended to be comprehensive or formalized, but rather to provide you with an updated understanding of what is known, what is not known (see Finding the Gap), and moreover, what methods have been taken to develop relevant knowledge. Be sure that you begin note taking as soon as you start to retrieve and read the literature, as this will assist you in recalling important ideas and associations (Pautasso, 2013). While different reviewers take varied approaches to this stage, you can begin to identify and refine search terms (Boland et al., 2017). Start by searching one or two databases with these terms and skim through some of the relevant articles. Often, hand searching or ancestry searching the reference lists of these highly relevant articles can point you toward a "scientific trail" (Conn et al., 2003). Be sure that at this point you are considering different types of available evidence (e.g., primary studies, reviews, grey literature, commentaries, letters to the editor, and perhaps conference proceedings; Boland et al., 2017; Conn et al., 2003).

As mentioned, while this is not necessarily a formalized process, it is important to maintain documentation in real time at each step along the way, tracking of the references retrieved and their sources. We recommend using a reference manager at this point. During this initial search, you will need to determine whether there is enough published literature to draw from to inform your review (Bolderston, 2008). It is critical that you keep track of the literature reviews that are already published that are directly or peripherally related to your topic area. Assess when those literature reviews were conducted and published, which databases were searched, which articles/data were synthesized, and the venues in which the articles were published. Existing literature reviews can be useful in identifying experts in your field (Fink, 2020); during this process, you might also attempt to connect with some of these experts, if they are willing and able to do so (Boland et al., 2017). We advise that you make this connection toward the end of the initial search, once you have thoroughly acquainted yourself with the span of the literature and generated specific and significant questions that you would like to discuss with a content expert.

Finding the Gap

After you have conducted your initial search, culled the most relevant articles, and apprised yourself of the current state of the science, you are now tasked with identifying what is *not known* within the general domain of your selected topic. Realizing this gap can shape understanding of how you can maximally contribute to your field. It is generally helpful to create a table to record and track any identified literature that has helped to determine and may eventually inform the filling of this gap. Some questions intended to help guide the assessment of the literature include: Who comprises the population? What are the sociodemographic characteristic trends (e.g., sex/gender, age, race, and ethnicity) and clinical characteristics of the population? Additional questions to further guide the assessment of the literature include: Which settings or environments are being examined (e.g., outpatient, inpatient, community), and what components of a study intervention or implementation are being evaluated? Once you have reviewed these and related questions, it may become obvious to you where the gaps in the literature exist.

DEFINING THE REVIEW PURPOSE

Now that you are acquainted with the depth and breadth of the literature, you can proceed confidently in defining the purpose of your review, which will be informed by the themes noted and gaps identified in the initial informal literature search. As you work to define the purpose of your review, you will be tasked with considering the interests and knowledge needs of specific target readerships, which may include valued stakeholders. For example, consider if your topic area is about sleep in the intensive care unit and the intended purpose of the review is to assess the available evidence regarding barriers and facilitators of quality overnight sleep among patients in intensive care units. Then, the readership will likely include healthcare providers and staff who work in an intensive care unit, hospital administrators, researchers interested in topics pertinent to critical care settings and/or sleep, and potentially patients and families. Also consider if the topic area is vaccination among pediatric patients and the purpose is to review available evidence regarding vaccination hesitancy, uptake, and adherence to recommended vaccination schedules in children under 12 years of age. Then, the audience is likely to include pediatric healthcare providers and staff, healthcare policy makers, public health practitioners and researchers with an interest in infectious diseases and vaccination, and potentially family members and caregivers of pediatric patients. Another example to consider is if the topic area is renal transplantation and the purpose is to review existing literature investigating the efficacy of interventions to improve renal transplant outcomes. Then, the readership likely includes transplant providers and staff, researchers focused on transplant, patients who have or will undergo transplant, patient families and caregivers, and/or insurance agencies. Having a sense of the reason(s) why you are conducting a literature review, as well as the readership for whom you are writing, will help you to determine the scope of your review, the focus of your review purpose and question, and the structure of your process.

FORMULATING THE REVIEW QUESTION

Once you have completed your initial informal literature search that led to the defining of your topic area, you are now poised to formulate your review question (Boland et al., 2017). Formulating the review question entails a process of translating a general selected topic or problem area into a formal review question, which may involve your personal interests or concerns (Machi & McEnvoy, 2016) and is informed by your review purpose. Review question formulation is a pivotal step, as literature reviews are generally question-led (Booth et al., 2016). Indeed, formulating a specific and clear review question is arguably the most important step within the literature review and synthesis process (Souza et al., 2010), as it is a precisely stated question that guides the review and determines which data sources are eligible for inclusion (Souza et al., 2010). Depending on the nature of your topic area and defined review purpose, you may take different approaches to review question formulation. There are a multitude of different frameworks available to provide guidance for developing a question for a literature review. Here we provide an overview of several frameworks for question formulation, including PICO, PICo, PEO, PerSPecTIF, SPICE, and SPIDER (Table 3.4). If one of these

TABLE 3.4 LITERATURE REVIEW QUESTION FRAMEWORKS

PICO(TS) ■ Patient/Problem/Population ■ Intervention ■ Comparison/Control ■ Outcome(s) ■ Time (optional) ■ Study (optional)	PICo ■ Population/Problem ■ (Phenomena of) Interest ■ Context
PEO ■ Population ■ Exposure ■ Outcomes	PerSPECTiF ■ Perspective ■ Setting ■ Phenomenon of Interest/Problem ■ Environment ■ Comparison (optional) ■ Time/Timing ■ Findings
SPICE ■ Setting ■ Perspective ■ Intervention/Interest ■ Comparison ■ Evaluation	SPIDER ■ Sample ■ Phenomenon of Interest ■ Design ■ Evaluation ■ Research Type

frameworks does not fit your defined review purpose or anticipated approach to your review, then you may find it useful to explore which question frameworks have been previously used to guide reviews similar in topic or purpose to your own (University Libraries, University of Maryland, 2019).

The most commonly used framework to guide formulation of a quantitative literature review question is **PICO** (Booth et al., 2016; Eden et al., 2011; Higgins et al., 2019). All **PICO** frameworks have the same first four components: **P** represents the patient, problem, or population under study; **I** represents the intervention that is being examined; **C** represents the comparison, or intervention, for example a placebo, "usual care," active, or attentional control group; **O** represents the dependent variable, the outcome(s). Additional iterations of **PICO** include the **PICOT** and **PICOS** frameworks. In the **PICOTS** frameworks, the **T** represents time and the **S** represents the study type; limiting the time period during which studies are conducted and published and the methodologies used can help to limit the number of records eligible for inclusion in a review (Booth et al., 2016). Social interventions may be particularly affected by the context in which the intervention is delivered (Booth et al., 2016; Petticrew & Roberts, 2006). Cochrane Reviews defines the steps in a literature review in which the **PICO** framework can be used (Higgins et al., 2019). First, the **PICO** can be used during the protocol development stage to help determine eligibility criteria. Second, the **PICO** can be used during the synthesis stage to provide parameters for the synthesis. Third, the **PICO** of the included data sources represents what was explored in those studies.

Certain question frameworks are designed specifically for qualitative literature reviews and syntheses, which generally focus on understanding phenomena. In the **PICo** framework, **P** represents the population, **I** represents the phenomenon of interest, and **Co** represents the context of the study (Boland et al., 2017; Lockwood et al., 2020). **PEO** is another qualitative framework where **P** represents the population and the problem, **E** represents the exposure, and **O** represents the outcomes or themes (Bettany-Saltikov & McSherry, 2016). The **SPICE** framework focuses on the perspectives held by the population of interest and is particularly useful in exploring qualitative questions. In the **SPICE** framework, **S** represents setting, **P** represents perspective, **I** represents both the intervention and interest, **C** represents the comparison, and **E** represents evaluation (Booth et al., 2019; Higgins et al., 2019). Although new, **PerSPECTiF** is a promising extended framework that addresses complex interventions that are synthesized qualitatively (Booth et al., 2019). **Per** represents perspective, **S** represents setting, **P** represents the phenomenon of interest or problem, **E** represents environment, **C** represents comparison (which is optional), **Ti** represents time or timing, and **F** represents the findings. Further testing of this framework is recommended (Booth et al., 2019). **SPIDER** is another framework that can be used to guide qualitative review question formulation, **S** represents the sample, **P** represents the phenomenon of interest, **D** represents the design of the study, **E** represents the evaluation, and **R** represents the research type (Cooke et al., 2012; Higgins et al., 2019). While this is not an exhaustive overview of all frameworks available to formulate review questions, these frameworks provide a sense of the components to consider when formulating a quantitatively oriented, qualitatively oriented, or mixed methods (or other type of) review question.

The way in which you formulate your review question will significantly impact eligibility criteria, and therefore the literature included, and subsequently the results generated by your review and synthesis. The level of detail provided in each element of your review question will in part determine how general or specific your literature search will be. That is, how you define the relevant participants, interventions (or assessments), and outcomes, will ultimately inform your eligibility (inclusion/exclusion) criteria and therefore literature that is ultimately included in your review. For instance, if you are formulating a **PICO** question to evaluate the efficacy of home-based interventions in patients who have experienced a cerebrovascular accident (stroke), if you limit the age range of your patients to adults between 50 and 70 years of age, home-based nursing interventions only, the comparison (e.g., no home-based nursing), the outcome of interest (e.g., blood pressure control), your search will likely yield a small number of results, given the restrictions. However, if you include, for instance, patients of all ages, any home-based intervention (e.g., nursing, physical therapy, occupational therapy, speech and language therapy), and consider a range of outcomes (e.g., improvement in functional abilities, independence in activities of daily living, emergency department/acute care service use), you will likely locate and include a far greater number of data sources. That said, it requires a refined question to retrieve precisely the results that are true to your original purpose, sensitive, and specific. Formulating a review question that is both precise and appropriately broad allows one to not restrict to the point of few data thwarting a meaningful synthesis, while also not loosening criteria to the point of unfocused dissimilarity, which is equally difficult to synthesize.

CHOOSING THE OPTIMAL LITERATURE REVIEW AND SYNTHESIS TYPE

Once the review question has been formulated, the work of choosing the optimal literature review and synthesis type becomes a much easier task. When surveying possible types of reviews to conduct, initially the reviewer is advised to include only the review types that are appropriate for the specific review question. If you are a student, the course syllabus may require a specific type of review, for instance a narrative or scoping review. If the student is conducting a review for a thesis or dissertation, we suggest that there be a careful review of available guidelines and the criteria used to determine how the review will be assessed in regard to their requirements, and also discussed with an academic advisor. A student may follow specific organizational guidelines that provide direction on the allowable literature review types. For instance, if a reviewer submits a peer-reviewed protocol and is committed to conducting a Cochrane review or Joanna Briggs Institute review, then the type of review will be established and informed by existing organizational guidelines. If a reviewer is conducting a review to inform guidelines for a national or international organization, the organization will likely have expectations regarding the type of review that is required or recommended. For health policy professionals, a review may be guided by regulations or recommendations of the governmental and non-governmental agencies or other stakeholders that will be most impacted by the findings of the literature review.

Peer-reviewed journal guidelines may also influence the type of literature review that you choose to conduct, as only certain review types may be considered for publication in select journals. Particularly if a reviewer is considering a high impact factor journal for publication of their review, we recommend becoming familiar with the types of reviews that are most commonly published in that journal, as well as the guidelines and formatting requirements for submitting completed reviews for consideration for publication. However, accounting for certain journal specifications may be somewhat risky, as typically there is no guarantee that the review will be published in a specific target journal once it is completed and submitted.

DETERMINING WHEN AN ORIGINAL REVIEW REQUIRES UPDATING

There are times when a reviewer may choose not to complete a new review, but rather to update an existing original review of a related or the same topic of interest. The decision to update an existing review may occur after the reviewer has selected the topic area, completed an initial informal literature search, determined the intended review purpose, and formulated the review question. At this point, the reviewer may discover a similar review to what they were proposing, and also recognize that the review synthesis is missing more recently available literature. In situations in which there is significant overlap between your selected or intended review topic area and already published reviews, there may be an opportunity to approach the topic from a new angle. Possibilities to consider include updating an existing review with articles that have been released since the publication of the review, attempting to address the previous review limitations, or expanding upon earlier conclusions and syntheses with new perspectives (Pautasso, 2013).

This opportunity is partly why it is invaluable to familiarize yourself with the literature that is relevant to your review topic, purpose, and question—to avoid redundancy and to build upon existing scientific understanding, rather than reiterate what is already known. Alternatively, a reviewer may be an expert in a topic area and feel invested in ensuring that a review is updated in order to inform best clinical practice and/or policy. In this case, if possible, we recommend first connecting with the authors of the original review to determine their plans for future updates, interest in collaboration, or other recommendations.

There are several factors to consider when contemplating undertaking an update of an original review. The first is the age or date of publication of the original review. While age itself is an insufficient reason to update a review, the reviewer should consider changes that have occurred, or valuable literature that has been published since the original review was conducted and published. One change may be major differences in standards of care, informed by studies completed and published since the publication of the original review. Newer studies may be more comprehensive, may have used additional measures which may have a higher level of accuracy and sophistication, investigate novel interventions and implementation methods, and/or address relevant outcomes. Further, older original reviews may not have included all aspects of reviews or critical appraisal of the included literature; thus, all eligible data sources may have been included and synthesized to generate findings without exclusion of any studies. The reviewer may want to explore the topic or question of an original review from a different angle—perhaps more broadly, or more narrowly but with greater depth on one particular component. Also, the reviewer may want to complete and contribute the results of a meta-analysis for instance, if only a narrative synthesis was completed in an original systematic review.

As a reviewer becomes an expert in a topic area, the reviewer may choose to explore a sub-topic or a specialized domain within this topic area from a vantage point different than previously reviewed. For instance, a psychiatric nurse may be interested in the use of selective serotonin reuptake inhibitors in the setting of obsessive compulsive disorder; while a review may have been completed on outcomes of selective serotonin reuptake inhibitors in depression, anxiety, and post-traumatic stress disorder. While there is overlap in the intervention, the population of interest and controls/comparators differ. While similar in topic, the psychiatric nurse's proposed review has a different purpose, and the review will provide answers to a previously unanswered question. The related original review will undoubtedly provide a foundation for what existing studies have been included in a related but not identical synthesis and original review recommendations for future research.

WRITING THE REVIEW PROTOCOL

Review protocols are developed prior to commencing the review, specifying the review plan and ensuring that the review is thoughtfully planned and explicitly documented (Aromataris, 2020; Cochrane Library, 2021; Moher et al., 2015; National Institute for Health Research, 2021; Whittemore, 2005). The review protocol details the rationale for conducting the review and the a priori methodological and analytical approach; a detailed plan for the review that outlines and specifies the central objectives, concepts, and methods in advance of conducting the review (Littell et al., 2008), including eligibility criteria for primary studies (Whittemore, 2005). By developing a protocol prior to literature searching, data collection, and extraction, bias in the collection, extraction, and interpretation of findings can be minimized. The protocol signals to its reader that a review was conducted in a manner consistent with the original plan, and there was thus a level of accountability, expectation of research integrity, and full transparency carried throughout and following the literature review and synthesis process. Ideally, the protocol reduces random or unplanned decisions through the advance planning for anticipated problems. When the review is published, readers can follow and evaluate the reviewer's steps in accordance with the review protocol (Littell et al., 2008). The review protocol allows a reader to locate any potential deviations from the original plan and determine whether these deviations were influential in introducing bias and unexpected results at any level (Moher et al., 2015).

There are standard protocol components that are generally required and others that are recommended, as noted in Box 3.3. Dependent on the venue in which a reviewer intends to publish their protocol, there may be variance in the order, amount of information, and level of detail required and recommended. The cover page and other initial steps to the review protocol will contain the title, the team members, their location(s)/institutional affiliations, and possibly a relevant citation. The background includes the rationale and sets the stage for the remainder of the protocol. The objective includes the purpose of the review, with the rationale or justification as to why this review adds value to the scientific literature. The protocol may require the detailing of a review question, information on what population is being studied, the intervention and control groups for quantitative reviews/phenomena of interest for qualitative reviews, and the outcome(s) of interest. Eligibility criteria can be partialized into several components, such as timeframe, languages, and population of interest. A search strategy may also be required including information about which databases will be searched using which terminology. Details on the title/abstract and full text screening phases is provided, along with information on the investigators responsible for the screening, and whether screening will be completing independently by each of the two reviewers at each level; a plan for disagreement resolution between the two reviewers (e.g., identified third-party dispute mediator) will be described. The data extraction process will be detailed, again noting if this will be completed independently by each of the two reviewers. The tools that will be used for data extraction will also be delineated. The critical appraisal or quality assessment tools and process may be described, also noting if critical appraisal and quality assessment will be completed independently by each of the two reviewers. After this point, the reviewers will describe how they plan to extract, analyze, and synthesize the data, and the tools and/or strategies that they will use for this process (e.g., software/electronic platforms, home-grown tables, hand coding). Other review details may be required in the protocol. For example, conflicts of interest may be required, and acknowledgments of others who will contribute to the review as well as funding sources may be included. The current stage of the review (e.g., not yet started) may also be required to confirm that data extraction or an earlier phase of the review has not yet occurred.

Determination of where to publish the protocol is important to establish early. Review protocols are required by organizations that focus on the production of systematic and other types of literature reviews. With these types of organizations, software is typically provided to guide the protocol process that can provide a smooth transition for conducting and completing the literature review (Aromataris, 2020; Cochrane Library, 2021). Additionally, if the reviewer is writing a review within the context of a global literature review organization, the venue for publication of the protocol of that review will likely be predetermined. However, if the reviewer is independently completing a literature review, the reviewer is advised to consider the optimal venue for publication of the protocol. Potential venues for publication of a review protocol include PROSPERO, which is based in the United Kingdom, and is an international registry for systematic reviews (National Institutes of Health, 2021). BMC Systematic Reviews also publishes protocols (BioMed Central, 2020). Additionally, there are other journals that publish review protocols, which can be located in electronic databases including PubMed, Scopus, CINAHL, and other databases related to your topic area.

FORMING A REVIEW TEAM

A rigorous review cannot be completed in isolation. Thus, it is imperative that you thoughtfully and intentionally identify and recruit potential collaborators. Teams with in-depth expertise are typically interdisciplinary and bring together diverse skills and knowledge areas (Boland et al., 2017; Eden et al., 2011; Littell et al., 2008). As discussed earlier in this chapter, it is imperative that all selected team members have the available time, interest, and expertise in the topic, purpose, and question of the review. As conducting a literature review and synthesis is a lengthy and often time-consuming undertaking, it is important that all review team members demonstrate a strong commitment to remaining engaged with the review through to completion. Without this commitment, the literature review process can be slowed, contributing to an outdating of the review content that is not disseminated in a timely manner. If and when this happens, reviewers become required to either update the review from the point that they lasted collected data, or start the review again from the early stages. Both of these are outcomes that often leave review teams frustrated. In this situation, not only does the review potentially remain incomplete, but the science suffers because the review never gets to the point of dissemination. At the outset, clearly setting expectations for roles and levels of participation within the review team is vital to success. The possible roles that certain members of a review team may assume are outlined in Table 3.5. The role

TABLE 3.5 MEMBERS OF THE REVIEW TEAM

Role	Contribution
Primary reviewer	▪ Leads the team in the conduct of the review across all stages of the process, guiding decision-making. ▪ Offers methodological and/or content expertise.
Secondary reviewer	▪ Is involved in all stages of the review, under the leadership and guidance of the primary reviewer, supplementing the decision-making of the primary reviewer. ▪ Offers methodological and/or content expertise.
Medical librarian (*optional, strongly recommended*)	▪ Leads the development of the search strategy and execution of the search across electronic and other databases, under the leadership and guidance of the primary reviewer (and sometimes Secondary Reviewer).
Methodological expert (*optional*)	▪ Provides guidance regarding the review design, proper execution of sequential steps, including screening of records, data extraction, and data synthesis.
Content expert (*optional*)	▪ Offers additional content expertise, sharing insight into defining the purpose, formulating the question, and, importantly, data synthesis.
Other team members (*optional*)	▪ May serve as a mediator for disagreement resolution between the primary and secondary reviewers. ▪ May assist with the compilation and organization of data, as well as overall review and synthesis.

that each team member plays, and moreover, the degree of effort extended should be reflected in authorship, specifically author order. We recommend that you discuss authorship guidelines and expectations with each member of your review team prior to collectively undertaking any actions toward the literature review. When discussed early and upfront, you are more likely to avoid confusion and feelings of inequity around the time of submission for publication. If a contributor has consulted on only one small part of the review, then this person may ask to be placed in acknowledgments instead of having authorship. Many journals now have strict requirements about who can be included as an author on a review article, depending on the level of contribution to the review process and manuscript preparation.

The primary reviewer is considered the lead reviewer and is responsible for coordinating the roles of fellow review team members, providing oversight on the review process in its entirety. It is the primary reviewer's responsibility to establish a reasonable timeline for each review phase and completion with review team members, as well as to identify and recruit team members with specific expertise as needed. The primary reviewer is involved in each stage of the literature review. The secondary reviewer is also typically involved in each stage of the review, but under the leadership and direction of the primary reviewer. The secondary reviewer is a critical team member, as they need to be equipped to independently assess titles/abstracts and full texts, as well as independently complete data extraction, critical appraisals, and quality assessment of each data source. Two members are the minimum needed to complete a double or dual screening (vs. single screening) review process. Medical librarians are also critical review team members, as they have vast knowledge of how to comprehensively yet specifically locate literature in databases with an optimized search strategy. Without the input of a medical librarian, review teams risk overlooking integral data sources because of how certain articles might be indexed, or due to unawareness of certain databases that may be pertinent to a particular literature review. Medical librarians are generally also experienced in preparing a PRISMA flow diagram, which conveys to the reader the number and names of databases searched, number of titles, abstracts and full texts screened (including grey literature and hand searching, as applicable), number of duplicates removed, and ultimately, the number of articles included versus excluded, detailing reasons for exclusion. For quantitative, qualitative, and mixed methods (among other types of) reviews, methodological expertise is often required, particularly to support new or novice reviewers in completing a rigorous meta-analysis or meta-synthesis. Content experts may also be helpful, particularly for reviewers who are new to a topic area or are exploring a purpose or question, which may involve complex consideration of new concepts or processes. In this situation, a review may consider a one-time consult with a content expert, rather than requesting this expert to formally join the review team. Additional team members may be recruited to assist with various components of the review, such as a research assistant who may help with the organization and storage of data, and potentially with writing certain components of the literature review manuscript. Depending on the writing skill level of the team, editorial assistance may be useful in preparation to submit and enhance likelihood of publication. We recommend that depending on the extent of the involvement of different team members, you may want to recognize them in the acknowledgment section of your final literature review manuscript, if they are not already an author. As always, every review team member is responsible for adhering to the ethics of authorship, basing authorship decisions on the standards outlined by the International Committee of Medical Journal Editors regarding the roles of authors and contributors (International Committee of Medical Journal Editors, 2020).

ACTIVITIES
Activity I

As a nurse or other healthcare or health policy professional, you decide that you want to explore the possibility of using a quantitative or a qualitative question to complete a review in your area of interest. To compare and contrast the two types of questions, you search the literature for both types of reviews.

1. Determine a topic area in which you are interested in conducting a literature review and synthesis.

2. Access two or three databases to locate a quantitative and a qualitative review relevant to your selected topic.

3. Identify the research questions that guided the literature reviews. Determine the question frameworks that were used to formulate each question. Compare the questions: What is similar and what is different?

4. Brainstorm different rationales for using a quantitative, qualitative, or mixed methods (or other type of) review fitting to your topic of interest. What are the potential benefits and disadvantages of each methodological approach?

Activity II

You are a reviewer who is studying the topic of resilience in children and would like to conduct a literature review in this general topic area. You have determined that the purpose of your review will be to characterize the state of the science regarding child behavioral health outcomes following a natural disaster. Your review question is investigating whether children under 12 years of age who were exposed to a natural disaster experience higher rates of behavioral issues in school than those who have not been exposed to a natural disaster. First, you prepare to a write a review protocol. First, quickly jot down notes (electronically or on paper) regarding what you intend to include in your protocol. Second, quickly locate two or three already published review protocols relevant to pediatric populations, natural disaster studies, and/or adverse childhood experiences. Here are a few suggestions for protocols:

1. A systematic review of creativity-based interventions to foster resilience in preschool children (Verger et al., 2019).
   www.crd.york.ac.uk/PROSPERO/display_record.php?RecordID=160848

2. Meta-ethnography of the concept of resilience among young adults exposed to adverse childhood experiences (Leung et al., 2022).

www.crd.york.ac.uk/PROSPERO/display_record.php?RecordID=104007

3. A systematic review of child resilience indicators in natural disaster situations (Mohammadinia et al., 2018).

www.crd.york.ac.uk/PROSPERO/display_record.php?RecordID=106114

Now that you have read the review protocols in this topic area, consider your unique angle or contribution—what you might add, change, or tailor in your own review protocol. Next, further refine your review protocol ideas based on these reflections.

SUMMARY POINTS

A review may be a component of graduation requirements for a student, the result of a clinical need to develop guidelines addressing a practice issue, or inspired by a health policy debate that requires action to change. Regardless of the reason or the rationale as to "why," the undertaking of a literature review and synthesis can be a daunting task for novice and expert reviewers alike. When a reviewer decides that there is an apparent need to conduct a literature review and synthesis, a series of steps is initiated which can be managed one at a time, beginning with determining the feasibility of making this substantial commitment.

- Making the commitment requires appraising and understanding the time and skills that are necessary for the successful completion of the review process. Understanding the "why" that drives the commitment is imperative to remaining fueled throughout the duration of the often challenging and time intensive review process.

- Multiple resources are needed to conduct a quality literature review. The reviewer needs to realistically assess how much time the review will likely require, the level of skill and expertise needed, and who might contribute as valuable review team members. Support from your institutions, such as information technology access and financial support, can also be helpful in ensuring timely and quality completion of a literature review.

- Selecting the topic area requires the reviewer to determine the scientific relevance, as well as their familiarity and vested interest in a given topic. After selecting the general topic area, the reviewer should pursue an initial informal literature search to examine the depth, breadth, and gaps in the existing literature.

- After selecting a topic area and initially searching the literature, the reviewer is poised to define the purpose of the review. The review purpose narrows the selected general topic area to focus on just one specific sub-domain. A clearly defined review purpose will lend itself to the formulation of a strong review question.

- The review question will guide the entirety of the review, substantially informing establishment of review eligibility criteria. How the reviewer formulates the review question shapes the literature retrieved, and ultimately, the results and conclusions drawn. There are different frameworks available to formulate the review question. Dependent on if the review will be a quantitative, qualitative, or mixed methods review (among other types), the question components can differ. Who is being studied, what is being studied, and how it is being studied are all addressed by a well-formulated review question.

- Determining which type of literature review and synthesis to conduct, can occur once the review purpose and question are clearly established. Resources available and organizational guidelines may influence the type of literature review and synthesis that is preferable or possible.

- When a reviewer finds a previously published original review that is similar in purpose or question to what the reviewer had intended to review, it is important to assess first if that review requires updating. A review may be eligible for updating because of its age, but equally important, because of substantive changes in the state of the science.

- The review protocol is a foundational document that provides detailed guidance for the conduct of a literature review. The review protocol provides a roadmap that documents the rationale and proper conduct for the review, allowing readers to follow each step of your literature review process.

- Forming a review team that is fully committed to the process and equipped with the necessary skills and expertise will help to ensure the successful and timely completion of the literature review and synthesis. While a primary reviewer and secondary reviewer are essential for a dual screening process, other interdisciplinary team members, including a medical librarian, are valuable to a quality, streamlined literature review and synthesis process and product.

REFERENCES

Aromataris, E., & Munn, Z. (2020). Chapter 1: JBI systematic reviews. In E. Aromataris, & Z. Munn (Eds.), *JBI manual for evidence synthesis*. JBI. https://synthesismanual.jbi.global. https://doi.org/10.46658/JBIMES-20-02

Benner, P. (2001). *From novice to expert: Excellence and power in clinical nursing practice, commemorative edition*. Prentice-Hall, Inc.

Bettany-Saltikov, J., & McSherry, R. (2016). *How to do a systematic literature review in nursing: A step-by-step guide* (2nd ed.). Open University Press.

BioMed Central. (2020). *BMC systematic reviews*. https://systematicreviewsjournal.biomedcentral.com/

Boland, A., Cherry, M. G., & Dickson, R. (2017). *Doing a systematic review: A student's guide* (2nd ed.). Sage.

Bolderston, A. (2008). Writing an effective literature review. *Journal of Medical Imaging and Radiation Sciences*, 39(2), 86–92. https://doi.org/S1939-8654(08)00057-X

Booth, A., Sutton, A., & Papaioannou, D. (2016). *Systematic approaches to a successful literature review* (2nd ed.). Sage.

Booth, A., Noyes, J., Flemming, K., Moore, G., Tuncalp, O., & Shakibazadeh, E. (2019). Formulating questions to explore complex interventions within qualitative evidence synthesis. *BMJ Global Health*, 4(Suppl. 1), e001107-2018-001107. https://doi.org/10.1136/bmjgh-2018-001107

Cochrane Library. (2021). *About cochrane reviews*. https://www.cochranelibrary.com/about/about-cochrane-reviews

Conn, V. S., Isaramalai, S. A., Rath, S., Jantarakupt, P., Wadhawan, R., & Dash, Y. (2003). Beyond MEDLINE for literature searches. *Journal of Nursing Scholarship: An Official Publication of Sigma Theta Tau International Honor Society of Nursing, 35*(2), 177–182. https://doi.org/10.1111/j.1547-5069.2003.00177.x

Cooke, A., Smith, D., & Booth, A. (2012). Beyond PICO: The SPIDER tool for qualitative evidence synthesis. *Qualitative Health Research, 22*(10), 1435–1443. https://doi.org/10.1177/1049732312452938

Cooper, H. (2017). *Research synthesis and meta-analysis: A step-by-step approach* (5th ed.). SAGE.

Cronin, P., Ryan, F., & Coughlan, M. (2008). Undertaking a literature review: A step-by-step approach. *British Journal of Nursing (Mark Allen Publishing), 17*(1), 38–43. https://doi.org/10.12968/bjon.2008.17.1.28059

Eden, J., Levit, L., Berg, A., Morton, S., & Committee on Standards for Systematic Reviews of Comparative Effectiveness Research, & Institute of Medicine (Eds.) (2011). *Finding what works in health care: Standards for systematic review.* Washington, D.C.: The National Academies Press.

Fink, A. (2020). *Conducting research literature reviews: From the internet to paper* (5th ed.). SAGE.

Hart, C. (2018). *Doing a literature review: Releasing the research imagination* (2nd ed.). SAGE.

Higgins, J. P. T., Thomas, J., Chandler, J., Cumpston, M., Li, T., Page, M. J., & Welch, V. A. (Eds.) (2019). *Cochrane handbook for systematic reviews of interventions.* www.training.cochrane.org/handbook

International Committee of Medical Journal Editors. (2020). *Defining the role of authors and contributors.* http://www.icmje.org/recommendations/browse/roles-and-responsibilities/defining-the-role-of-authors-and-contributors.html

Leung, D. Y. L., Chan, A. C. Y., & Ho, G. W. K. (2022). Resilience of emerging adults after adverse childhood experiences: A Qualitative Systematic Review. *Trauma Violence Abuse, 23*(1), 163–181. https://doi.org/10.1177/1524838020933865

Littell, J. H., Corcoran, J., & Pillai, V. (2008). *Systematic reviews and meta-analysis.* Oxford University Press.

Lockwood, C., Porrit, K., Munn, Z., Rittenmeyer, L., Salmond, S., Bjerrum, M., Loveday, H., Carrier, J., & Stannard, D. (2020). Chapter 2: Systematic reviews of qualitative evidence. In E. Aromataris, & Z. Munn (Eds.), *JBI manual for evidence synthesis.* JBI. https://synthesismanual.jbi.global. https://doi.org/10.46658/JBIMES-20-03

Machi, L. A., & McEnvoy, B. T. (2016). *The literature review: Six steps to success* (3rd ed.). Corwin.

Mohammadinia, L., Ardalan, A., Khorasani-Zavareh, D., Ebadi, A., Malekafzali, H., & Fazel, M. (2018). Domains and indicators of resilient children in natural disasters: A systematic literature review. *International Journal of Preventive Medicine, 9*, 54. https://doi.org/10.4103/ijpvm.IJPVM_1_18

Moher, D., Shamseer, L., Clarke, M., Ghersi, D., Liberati, A., Petticrew, M., Shekelle, P., Stewart, L. A., & PRISMA-P Group. (2015). Preferred reporting items for systematic review and meta-analysis protocols (PRISMA-P) 2015 statement. *Systematic Reviews, 4*, 1-4053-4-1. https://doi.org/10.1186/2046-4053-4-1

National Institute for Health Research. (2021). *PROSPERO, international prospective register of systematic reviews.* https://www.crd.york.ac.uk/PROSPERO/

Pautasso, M. (2013). Ten simple rules for writing a literature review. *PLoS Computational Biology, 9*(7), e1003149. https://doi.org/10.1371/journal.pcbi.1003149

Petticrew, M., & Roberts, H. (2006). *Systematic reviews in the social sciences: A practical guide.* Blackwell Publishing.

Souza, M. T., Silva, M. D., & Carvalho, R. (2010). Integrative review: What is it? How to do it? *Einstein (Sao Paulo, Brazil), 8*(1), 102–106. https://doi.org/10.1590/S1679-45082010RW1134

University Libraries, University of Maryland. (2019). *Framing a research question.* https://lib.guides.umd.edu/SR/research_question

Verger, N., McAloney-Kocaman, K., Thomson, J., & Guiller, J. (2019). *A systematic review of creativity-based interventions to foster resilience in preschool children* (CRD42019160848). PROSPERO. https://www.crd.york.ac.uk/prospero/display_record.php?ID=CRD42019160848

Whittemore, R. (2005). Combining evidence in nursing research: Methods and implications. *Nursing Research, 54*(1), 56–62. https://doi.org/00006199-200501000-00008

4

Searching the Literature

Susan W. Buchholz and Kirsten A. Dickins

A search strategy is a process that allows the reviewer to determine, at a precise level, how the reviewer will search the vast array of global literature when conducting a literature review and synthesis.

CHAPTER OUTLINE

- Objectives
- Preparing for the Literature Search
- Developing the Search Strategy
- Determining the Intent of the Literature Search
- Engaging the Literature Review Team in the Search Strategy Process
- Choosing the Search Terms
- Executing the Search Strategy
- Activities
- Summary Points
- References

At the time that you begin reading this chapter, you would have long since made the commitment to your literature review and synthesis. Following through on this, you have selected your topic area and conducted an initial informal literature search. These steps have together helped you to find the gap, establish your review purpose, formulate your review question, and write your protocol. Now it is time for you to develop and execute the search strategy. Developing and executing your formal search strategy will be a collaborative and iterative process on which the results of your literature review and synthesis largely rest. Ensuring the accuracy of your search strategy and the comprehensiveness of its execution is imperative to the precision of the results of your review and breadth of your synthesis.

LEARNING OBJECTIVES

In this chapter, we discuss the steps that are necessary to developing and executing a precise search strategy. By the end of this chapter, you will be able to:

- Describe how to prepare to strategically search the literature
- Develop an optimized search strategy
- Determine the intent of a literature search
- Identify which team members are vital to executing an optimized search strategy
- Select search terms to include in a search strategy, using MeSH and text words
- Recognize how to execute a search strategy

PREPARING FOR THE LITERATURE SEARCH

A comprehensive and accurate search of the literature is essential to obtaining valid results in your literature review and synthesis. Put otherwise, the results of your search will directly inform the conclusions that you draw in the context of your review and synthesis. Without a structured and comprehensive search, the results of your search may be biased and not representative of the depth and breadth of available knowledge. A literature search is not meant to locate only positive studies, though these may be overrepresented in published literature. A literature search is also not meant to only locate studies that are easy to find. Rather, it is incumbent upon you and your review team to uncover all evidence that is relevant to your review purpose and question (Cooper & Hedges, 2009). The conclusions that are reached after conducting a literature review are heavily impacted by various methodological factors, including the selected search criteria, terms, and literature sources (Dalton et al., 2016). If valid studies are not included in a literature review, then the review is inadequate and may be biased and may not be representative of the work that is globally available, resulting in potentially misinformed conclusions (Whittemore, 2005).

Being systematic is one process intended to help reduce the likelihood of bias and ensure comprehensive and efficient identification of all available literature (Booth et al., 2016). Being systematic begins by creating and leveraging a thoroughly considered and well-planned search strategy. The process of building your search strategy will be dynamic and iterative, requiring continuous assessment and refinement (Aromataris & Riitano, 2014). Thus, it is imperative that ample time to develop your search strategy is built into your literature review and synthesis timeline. This search strategy is the cornerstone of a well-conducted search that will identify relevant articles, and ultimately produce the highest quality results (Bolderston, 2008).

Document the Literature Search Process

As it will continue to be reiterated throughout this and subsequent chapters, it is essential to diligently document the selected search terms and process undertaken to curate

---

BOX 4.1   SEARCH STRATEGY STEPS

1. Determine the intent of the search
2. Engage the literature review team in the search strategy process
   - Consult with a medical librarian
   - Leverage key members of the literature review team
3. Choose the search terms
   - Early exploration of search terms
   - Medical Subject Headings (MeSH terms)
   - Text words and keywords
   - Determine search restrictions
4. Execute the search strategy
   - Review the search strategies rules
   - Use of Boolean operators and symbols
   - Search syntax
   - Electronic database searching
   - PubMed
   - Other types of searching
   - Searching the grey literature

---

your specific search strategy; tracking this process will allow for later replication of your search (Pautasso, 2013) by other reviewers, and/or your own review team in the case of a literature review update. Information technologies can aid reviewers by making each step in the literature process more transparent, efficient, and accessible.

DEVELOPING THE SEARCH STRATEGY

A search strategy is a process that allows the reviewer to determine, at a precise level, how they will search the vast array of global literature when conducting a literature review and synthesis. There are several steps involved in the search strategy process (see Box 4.1) including determining the intent of the search, engaging the review team in developing the search strategy, choosing the search terms, and executing the search strategy.

DETERMINING THE INTENT OF THE SEARCH

In setting out to create the search strategy, the review team benefits from first centering on the established intent of the search. The primary reviewer needs to be able to articulate the purpose and scope of the review with ease and clarity. For example, a scoping review may be used by the reviewer to clarify concepts, as well as to determine inclusion criteria and which questions should be asked in a later systematic review. In this case, a scoping review provides the reviewer with an opportunity to answer these precursor questions prior to engaging in a systematic review (Munn et al., 2018). When a reviewer conducts a comprehensive state-of-the-science review, an extensive search strategy will be necessary. Cochrane systematic reviews (Cochrane Library, 2020) and Joanna Briggs Institute systematic reviews (Joanna Briggs Institute, 2020) are examples of thoroughly completed literature reviews necessarily entailing detailed search strategies.

Regardless of the depth and breadth of the review, the reviewer needs to establish a clear review question that will provide guidance for determining search terms and search strategy parameters. A clear review question will drive the type of data that will be sought in the review. If the question is one that requires a qualitative answer, the reviewer will know to focus the search strategy on qualitative studies that have been completed on the topic of interest. If the review question is addressed primarily through randomized controlled trials, the reviewer will focus on locating clinical trials. However, if the question is best answered by including studies that use varied designs, the reviewer may consider conducting an integrative review, allowing for terminology relevant to different study designs to be included in the search.

The reviewer must also establish a baseline understanding of the available literature. In taking time to familiarize oneself with seminal literature in an area of interest, the reviewer will ensure that a similar review has not already been published. In this process, the reviewer will also locate informative articles and identify key relevant terms. While becoming acquainted with the literature, the reviewer should note the authors of relevant articles, the journals in which important articles are being published, and who is citing these data sources in which venues. Completing this early investigative work affords the reviewer an opportunity to survey the field of reviews and noteworthy articles that have been published on the topic of interest.

The following series of exhibits operationalizes the steps of the search strategy development and execution process. The series of exhibit boxes provide information for each respective step of this process through leveraging an exemplar of how a reviewer searches the literature when asking the question of *"What type of nursing interventions are most effective in improving infectious disease outcomes for aging women who have immigrated?"* Exhibit 4.1 determines the intent of the search.

EXHIBIT 4.1 DETERMINING THE INTENT OF THE SEARCH

A clinician/researcher is working in the area of providing care for aging women who have immigrated. The researcher is particularly concerned about what happens to members of this population when they are exposed to an infectious disease, as the researcher has noted in their own clinical work that the health outcomes for this population, especially women who are aging, can be poorer than women who have not immigrated.

(continued)

EXHIBIT 4.1 DETERMINING THE INTENT OF THE SEARCH (*continued*)

The researcher completes a preliminary search of the literature and notices that while there are several excellent key articles related to this area, there are no literature reviews that specifically address this topic. Several key articles include:

- Interventions to Improve Immigrant Health. A Scoping Review
  https://pubmed.ncbi.nlm.nih.gov/28339883/
- Health of Refugees and Migrants–Where Do We Stand and What Directions Should We Take?
  www.ncbi.nlm.nih.gov/pmc/articles/PMC6518249/
- A Rapid Review of Evidence-Based Information, Best Practices and Lessons Learned in Addressing the Health Needs of Refugees and Migrants
  www.who.int/migrants/publications/partner-contribution_review.pdf

The reviewer develops a working question "What type of nursing interventions are most effective in improving infectious disease outcomes for aging women who have immigrated."
The researcher also develops a PICO question for the review:

- P: Aging women who have immigrated
- I: Infectious disease nursing interventions
- C: No care or usual care
- O: Morbidity and mortality related to infectious diseases

Because they do not want to exclude any relevant work done in this area, the researcher determines that an integrative review approach would be appropriate – allowing them to include non-experimental, quasi-experimental, and experimental studies. The researcher determines that there will not be a start date, since they want to glean an accurate historical perspective on the topic from the literature. The researcher is only fluent in English, so limits the search to English. However, it may be helpful if there is access to colleagues who may be fluent in other languages, given the likelihood that articles may be written in languages other than English.

ENGAGING THE LITERATURE REVIEW TEAM IN THE SEARCH STRATEGY PROCESS

At this point, the primary reviewer has already engaged at least one content expert or learner who is invested in contributing to a successful literature review and synthesis. If the reviewer has not identified a content expert to participate in the literature review, we recommend at minimum, consulting with an expert who understands the intricacies of and/or has experience in conducting a literature review and synthesis.

Consult With a Medical Librarian

Ideally, a search strategy for a health-related literature review will be developed in consultation with an expert in the field of data retrieval. There are different professionals that have data retrieval expertise who may be known by different names, such as an information specialist, informationist, search coordinator, or most commonly, a librarian (e.g., medical librarian). In this chapter, the focus is on literature reviews that are relevant to healthcare system improvements. The term *medical librarian* will be used throughout this chapter to represent librarians with expertise in healthcare. Medical librarians have unique educational qualifications in library science and health information. While medical librarians are referenced most frequently here, keep in mind that the title of the expert with whom you consult may differ. Working closely with a medical librarian will allow you access to expertise in the complicated field of searching the vast literature. This is necessary when there is certain grammar and logic embedded in a quality search strategy (Fink, 2020), information of which you may not be aware, which is often best known by a medical librarian. If you are affiliated with a university, especially those connected to an academic medical center, there may be a dedicated medical librarian who is well versed in literature review techniques, including designing search strategies and executing searches. Further, your institution may offer tutorials on searching electronic databases and offer personalized assistance with designing and executing searches.

When a reviewer does not have access to an expert in health library science, it may be challenging to initially develop an adequately comprehensive search strategy. Both Cochrane Reviews and the National Academy of Medicine (formerly the Institute of Medicine) recommend using a medical librarian from the beginning of the design of the study protocol (Eden et al., 2011; Lefebvre et al., 2019). If possible, the reviewer should verify whether funding is available for a consultation with a medical librarian. Medical librarians who contribute substantially to literature review design, conceptualization, and execution may be considered as an author on a publication. It may also be helpful for an inexperienced reviewer to partner with a more experienced reviewer to develop the search strategy. Barring these options, we advise the reviewer to set aside time to learn the skills and techniques necessary to developing comprehensive search strategies; this is most efficiently done by identifying opportunities for practice.

Leveraging Key Members of the Literature Review Team

In addition to a medical librarian, the literature review team may need at least one additional team member. This team member will work closely with the primary reviewer and medical librarian to determine an optimal combination of words and databases that will comprehensively locate relevant literature that is pertinent to the review. Ideally, this third review team member should have expertise in the content matter that is being explored. Experts in methodology and statistical analyses (Eden et al., 2011) may need to be consulted at this stage to aid in determining precise and accurate search terms. For example, a methodologist might be asked to provide language when reviewing studies employing sequential multiple assignment randomized trial (SMART) designs, advising on use of terms such as initial or augmented interventions, whereas a statistician may be needed to advise on terminology such as odds ratio or forest plot or other meta-analysis related phrases. Exhibit 4.2 provides information on search strategy team development.

EXHIBIT 4.2 SEARCH STRATEGY TEAM DEVELOPMENT

The reviewer is already a clinician in the area of women's health and works in a clinic that provides care for older women who have immigrated. The reviewer is aware that they will need to work closely with a medical librarian to capture the global literature that will inform this topic.

The reviewer works in an institution that has a medical librarian with whom they can consult. The reviewer decides to invite the medial librarian to join the search strategy team.

The reviewer also determines that while they understand clinical practice in infectious diseases, they do not have the in-depth expertise of an infectious disease expert. Therefore, the reviewer seeks out a healthcare provider who has expertise in this area and is able to locate a healthcare provider who is an expert in gerontology and infectious diseases.

The reviewer sets a meeting with the medical librarian and the additional healthcare expert. They each determine the roles that they will have while searching the literature.

CHOOSING THE SEARCH TERMS

Choosing precise and accurate search terms is an imperative first step in ensuring that you will comprehensively locate relevant literature with the search strategy.

Early Exploration of Search Terms

As already noted, a carefully crafted review purpose and a well-specified review question are foundational to your search strategy (Fink, 2020). Leveraging some of the terms in the review question, you can begin branching out to consider other possible words and phrases that pertain to your selected review topic, including synonyms, and alternate terms (Bolderston, 2008; Cooper et al., 2018). There are a number of approaches to begin drafting this list; you might start by jotting down keywords, frequently occurring terms, or words associated with those that you routinely encountered while reading the articles retrieved in your initial literature search. You might reference previously published reviews with content relevant to your own review. Often, search strategies are available as online appendices, and in some cases, in the body of the manuscript. These developed and utilized search strategies can serve as both positive and negative examples; while you will not explicitly follow another search strategy, you might use these examples to formulate your ideas as to how to begin to approach developing your own search strategy, drawing from the strengths and addressing prior search strategy limitations.

Controlled Vocabularies

Controlled vocabularies are a searchable thesaurus, or collection of biomedical terms that are used to index, catalogue, and search biomedical databases. It is useful to use controlled vocabularies when they are available, as this provides improved searching functionality. Medical Subject Headings (MeSH) terms are one of the most popularly known controlled vocabularies, used for searching PubMed and Ovid MEDLINE. Another example of a controlled vocabulary is the Subject Heading List used to search EBSCO's CINAHL (www.connect.ebsco.com/s/article/CINAHL-Help-Sheet?language=en_US). The following examples and explanations will refer to using MeSH terms.

Each MeSH term represents a single concept in the biomedical literature. There are currently over 29,000 MeSH terms available (www.nlm.nih.gov/mesh/intro_preface.html#pref_rem), which are updated annually. MeSH terms are applied by indexers who read the articles that have recently been added to MEDLINE and tag each article with the appropriate MeSH terms. Then, when a user searches on a MeSH term, the articles that have been tagged with that MeSH term are retrieved.

To use MeSH terms, the reviewer can use the general MeSH website and enter related terms into the search box (www.ncbi.nlm.nih.gov/mesh). MeSH terms are arranged using hierarchical logical groupings with the broadest terms positioned highest and the more specific terms placed under the broader terms. Using MeSH terms provides a higher level of uniformity when indexing by subject, in contrast to non-standardized, more arbitrary uses of terminology.

If the term entered in a PubMed search box is a MeSH term, a search for that MeSH term will be automatically provided. There is information available on the National Library of Medicine's website regarding how to search for MeSH terms (MeSH browser) and ensure accurate MeSH phrasing (such as this tutorial: www.nlm.nih.gov/mesh/introduction.html). It is also helpful to consult a medical librarian for assistance with identifying the optimal MeSH terms for your literature search. For example, rather than search "American Indians"[MeSH] the correct MeSH term/phrasing is "Indians, North American"[MeSH]. The search term itself will consist of the MeSH term followed by [MeSH] or [mh]. For example, searching either "Deafness"[MeSH] or "Deafness" [mh] will return all articles tagged with the MeSH term "Deafness".

There are some caveats to these general principles. MeSH terms can require up to 6 months to be applied, so if your search relies exclusively on MeSH terms, you may not capture the most recently published articles. Also, MeSH terms are regularly updated and new terms are added to the MeSH vocabulary. However, existing articles are typically not retrospectively indexed. In other words, if a new term is added in 2021, while all articles added to PubMed after 2021 will likely be tagged with the new MeSH term, articles published earlier than 2021 will likely not be retrospectively tagged with this MeSH term and therefore potentially missed in your search. Additionally, identifying

---

EXHIBIT 4.3 EXAMPLE OF MeSH TERM USAGE

There is a MeSH term for the selected population: "Emigrants and Immigrants."

This MeSH term is defined as "People who leave their place of residence in one country and settle in a different country." To conduct a search using this MeSH term, you would include it in your search strategy: "Emigrants and Immigrants" [MeSH].

There is also a potentially relevant sub-category for this MeSH term: "Undocumented Immigrants." Unless otherwise specified, searching for "Emigrants and Immigrants" will include the sub-category: "Undocumented Immigrants." If the reviewer wants to exclude "Undocumented Immigrants," they would search "Emigrants and Immigrants"[mh:noexp] which stands for "MeSH, not exploded."

This specific MeSH term was introduced in 2008. This means that no citations prior to 2008 will be retrieved by a search that includes only this MeSH term. For this reason, the search strategy should include the keywords (emigrant* OR immigrant*) for comprehensiveness of historical perspective.

---

the proper MeSH term to use may not be immediately obvious. For example, there are separate MeSH terms for "Anxiety" and "Anxiety Disorders" and an experienced librarian can help you choose the most appropriate term specific to your review. Additionally, indexers at the National Library of Medicine may apply a MeSH term that varies slightly from the MeSH term that you intended, you may apply an incorrect MeSH term, or you might overlook a MeSH term altogether. For these reasons, a complete search strategy includes both MeSH terms and non-MeSH keywords. It is generally advisable to use the MeSH term itself as one of the keywords. For example, an optimized search might include these terms: "Deafness"[MeSH] OR deaf* OR "hearing loss".

An example of application of a MeSH term follows, pertaining specifically to *pressure ulcers*. Articles written about *pressure ulcers* may use the terms *pressure ulcers* (which is a MeSH term), or *pressure sores, HAPU* (Hospital Acquired Pressure Ulcers), or simply *bedsores*, among other potential terms. To retrieve articles that use any of these keywords, a reviewer must search each of these terms. All articles that use any of these terms should be tagged with the MeSH term "Pressure Ulcer"; ideally, using the single MeSH term will return all articles that use any of the various terms mentioned. However, there is a possibility that as discussed, MeSH term tagging did not occur with absolute precision; hence, it is important to use a comprehensive search strategy employing both MeSH terms and non-MeSH terms alike.

Exhibit 4.3 provides an example of a specific MeSH term that can be used in the exemplar.

Text Words and Keywords

Although it is preferable to leverage the use of MeSH terms whenever possible, the precise term or phrase that is sought may not be available through the National Library of Medicine. If this is the case, the reviewer needs to generate their own additional search terms, sometimes referred to as *text words* or *keywords*. Text words or keywords are the terms or phrases that are used in a search strategy to retrieve relevant literature from diverse data sources (Bolderston, 2008; Fink, 2020). In this situation, the reviewer may choose to identify text words or keywords that involve the topic as it is commonly discussed in the literature, as noted during the initial literature review. Alternate spellings of particular terms and phrases must also be considered when selecting text words or keywords (Bolderston, 2008); that is, there may be different ways to spell or display relevant concepts, particularly in different versions of the English language. It is incumbent upon the reviewer to note all potential spellings of the same text word or keyword so that alternate possibilities can be incorporated into the search strategy. One way to refine a text word or keyword search is to limit the fields in which the text word appears. For example, in PubMed, a reviewer can limit results to those in which the desired text words or keywords appear in only the title or abstract fields. Delimiting the potential fields can aid in refining the search results to those that are the most fitting.

Determine Search Restrictions

Your search strategy will involve certain purposeful restrictions that should reflect your intended outcomes. If no restrictions are applied, results retrieved will likely be unfocused and unwieldy. Applying search restrictions necessarily entails awareness and accurate reflection of your eligibility criteria. Examples of purposeful restrictions include those pertaining to the age or gender of the population that you wish to understand. If the author is able to read articles in only one language, and no one else on the review team can assist with fluent language interpretation, you will likely need to limit the review to one language. However, it is important to recognize that articles pertinent to your topic area may be written in other languages and not translated into English; it is thus beneficial to determine in advance how these articles will be handled, so that pertinent literature is not unnecessarily excluded. If you choose to exclude this literature, we recommend that if this is a challenge that you encounter in your review, include this language restriction as a limitation in your final review and synthesis.

Year of publication may also be restricted by specifying a timeframe for publication, or publication start and/or end date (Bolderston, 2008). For instance, if there is a vast amount of literature published over the past several decades, there may have been substantive changes in the field that render the earlier literature less relevant or irrelevant; in this situation, the reviewer may want to limit the time frame, excluding outdated, earlier literature. Alternatively, the reviewer may limit the timeframe if published literature reviews have already included the literature up to a certain year; the review update may thus include literature only after this point. However, as the reviewer determines the timeframe, it is imperative to ensure that timeframe limitations are applied to all databases. In preparing for future publication, it is also helpful to be aware of papers in press (Pautasso, 2013).

Depending on the type of literature review, you may limit your search by article type and type of primary source (Galvan & Galvan, 2017). You may also limit by study design, such as using only randomized controlled trials or using only a specific qualitative methodology. If you are conducting an umbrella review, you may search only for literature reviews. In a narrative review or integrative review, you might include professional practice standard reports or may limit by the funding source type (Fink, 2020). PubMed provides filters that allow you to limit your search. For example, you can limit by publication date or language. However, the filters for population age and gender should be used with caution if you are conducting a truly comprehensive search. These are MeSH terms, and the caveats listed previously apply here as well. The limitations for a complete search strategy will include both PubMed filters and appropriate keywords.

Use of Boolean Operators and Symbols

Boolean algebra is a building block of many digital applications and is an important concept in database searching. Boolean algebra was developed by George Boole, an English mathematician in the 19th century (Britannica, The Editors of Encyclopaedia, 2021). Boolean logic is used to establish relationships between keywords or concepts while searching, using tools called Boolean operators.

Common Boolean operators include AND, OR, and NOT. Less common Boolean operators include NEAR or ADJ (adjacent). Boolean operators should be typed in capitalized letters. Words used to return articles about the same topic, whether MeSH terms or keywords, should be combined using OR within a single set of parentheses. For example, (Aged[MeSH] OR aged OR geriatric OR elderly) will return articles that were tagged with the MeSH term "Aged" OR that have the words "aged," "geriatric," or "elderly" as keywords. Using parentheses allows for the databases to understand the order of operations. Much like the math you learned in grade school, computations within parentheses are done first. For example $(7 + 2) \times 5$ will produce a different result than $7 + (2 \times 5)$.

Let us say that you are searching for literature addressing bruising in the aging populations. Your initial search strategy may look something like the following:

- (Aged [MeSH] OR aged OR geriatric OR elderly)
- AND ("Contusions"[MeSH] OR contusions OR bruises OR ecchymosis)

To fully comprehend and apply Boolean logic with the use of Boolean operators, it may help to think of the logic in everyday terms. A commonly understood example of Boolean logic in practice is that of online shopping. Let us use the example of online shopping for shoes for an upcoming event. You may visit a given store's website and search and specify that you are shopping for shoes, and in some instances, a specified gender. You select a size, perhaps a style preference, and likely a color preference. Your online shoe search, using Boolean logic, looks like the following search string: Women (or Men) AND (8 OR 8.5 OR [another size]) AND (rounded toe loafer OR pointed toe pump) AND (black OR silver OR [another color]). A Boolean search string, such as the aforementioned example, can be modified. Say you notice a color option "metallic." You decide that you would be happy with gold or silver or metallic, so you adapt your selected color preferences accordingly. Now, your Boolean search string includes "metallic" and the color preference component of the string now reads: (black OR silver OR metallic). You can further restrict your shoe search, for example, by limiting to a few favorite bands or a preferred material, adding to the search string: (Brand X OR Brand Y) AND (microfiber OR cotton).

Additional Search Symbols and Operators

Besides Boolean operators, a few additional symbols can be used to adjust search results. For example, if a reviewer wants to search for the various forms/suffixes of a root word, an asterisk (*) is generally used to facilitate this truncation. The truncation option may be used when there are various spellings or forms of the latter part of the word, or if the reviewer wants to include singular and plural words that begin with the same letter(s) (e.g., orthop* returns the terms orthopedic, orthopedics, orthopaedic, orthopaedics, etc.). Wildcards are used to represent any character within a word and is typically represented by a pound symbol (#), with each # symbol representing 0–1 characters. However, different databases can use different symbols for their wildcards. For example, searching on "behavio#r" is effective in CINAHL but not in PubMed.

Search Syntax

After MeSH terms and text words have been carefully chosen by the literature review team, a decision needs to be made as to how to use Boolean operators to optimize the search to retrieve relevant articles and exclude irrelevant records. Medical librarians have expertise in translating the search string between databases, or in other words, selecting database indexing terms and combining search terms (Cooper et al., 2018). Each database requires creating a different search syntax, dependent on each respective set of database rules.

Using as an example the chapter exemplar, Exhibit 4.4 shows how the reviewer can determine the beginning steps of the search strategy query in PubMed.

EXHIBIT 4.4 DECIDING ON A SEARCH STRATEGY FOR PUBMED

The research team develops a search strategy for their literature review, using the PICO format as a guide. They discuss which words to use for women, aging, immigration/immigrants, infectious disease, and nursing.

For gender, the team decides to use "Women"[MeSH] OR "Female"[MeSH]. They include keywords women OR woman OR female. They consider "mother" or "daughter" and decide to search on "mother" as they are focusing on aging women.

(continued)

EXHIBIT 4.4 DECIDING ON A SEARCH STRATEGY FOR PUBMED (*continued*)

This part of the search string appears as: "Women"[MeSH] OR "Female"[MeSH] OR women OR woman OR female OR mother.

When they examine aging they find the MeSH term of "Aged"[MeSH]. They note that this term refers to a person who is 65 to 79 years of age. There is a MeSH term "Aged, 80 and over"[MeSH] that is also available. Therefore, they determine to use both terms. They also add on the words (OR aged OR geriatric* OR elderly), resulting in the following search string:

- "Aged"[MeSH] OR "Aged, 80 and over"[MeSH] OR aged OR geriatric* OR elderly

For immigration/immigrants, they determine that they will use this word sequence: "Emigrants and Immigrants"[MeSH] OR (emigrant* OR immigrant*). They include the concept of "Refugee" as both a MeSH term and a keyword.

- "Emigrants and Immigrants"[MeSH] OR emigrant* OR immigrant* OR "Refugees"[MeSH] OR refugees

With infectious diseases, they determine that "Communicable diseases"[MeSH] is a term that is inclusive of locating studies that examine infectious diseases. They also add on (OR infection*)

- "Communicable diseases"[MeSH] OR "communicable diseases" OR infecti*

For nursing, they will use the term "Nursing"[MeSH]. They also add NOT "Breast feeding"[MeSH] as this term can be seen when using the word nursing, which can have multiple meanings.

- ("Nursing"[Mesh] OR Nurs*) NOT "Breast feeding"[MeSH]

A final search strategy may look like this:
(((("Women"[MeSH] OR "Female"[MeSH] OR women OR woman OR female OR mother)
AND ("Aged"[MeSH] OR "Aged, 80 and over"[MeSH] OR aged OR geriatric* OR elderly))
AND ("Emigrants and Immigrants"[MeSH] OR emigrant* OR immigrant* OR "Refugees"[MeSH] OR refugees))
AND ("Communicable diseases"[MeSH] OR "communicable diseases" OR infecti*))
AND (("Nursing"[MeSH] OR Nurs*) NOT "Breast feeding"[MeSH])
Using PubMed, the reviewers apply these word choices through several different scenarios, using only a couple of them in combination (yielding thousands of results), to using them all in combination (yielding far fewer results).

Working with the medical librarian, they eventually agree on a search strategy to query PubMed. They are also aware that search queries will be tailored uniquely for different databases.

EXECUTING THE SEARCH STRATEGY

The steps entailed in developing and executing your search will be presented in the methods section of your literature review and synthesis manuscript, allowing readers to follow your course of action as well as assess for any potential bias. Additionally, providing information regarding the databases accessed, search terms/strategy, inclusion and exclusion criteria, and publication date parameters, will add objectivity to your conclusions (Liumbruno et al., 2013). Systematic reviews should include a reproducible search strategy (PRISMA, 2021). You may choose to or be asked to publish the precise syntax for your search strategy—including search terms, MeSH terms, text words, and Boolean operators—precisely as they were entered during the database search. Even if you do not publish the precise syntax of the search strategy, it can be helpful to provide at least an outline of the terms that you searched (MeSH and non-MeSH), and a description of how you combined the search terms. In so doing, readers will be able to review your terms, and if they choose to do so, replicate your search.

Review the Search Strategies

Each electronic database outlines unique rules regarding how to execute a search. While a reviewer can enter words into a database search box and review the results retrieved, the publications retrieved will likely be limited and not comprehensively reflective of the original literature review question and may retrieve unrelated articles. It is worth the reviewer's time to read and closely follow the instructions and video tutorials regarding how to conduct a search within each respective database.

Electronic Database Searching

Once your search strategy is finalized, either a medical librarian or the primary reviewer will execute the search (Boland et al., 2017). Contemporary literature searches are conducted electronically in most universities, academic medical centers, and health facilities. The search accuracy is maximized by tailoring and executing the search in multiple electronic databases. Informal criteria for determining which and how many (total number of) electronic databases that your review team searches is detailed in the following paragraphs. It is recommended that you use at minimum two or three highly credible databases, which exclusively include high-quality publications with updated data (Liumbruno et al., 2013). However, if you are conducting a highly comprehensive literature search attempting to yield a maximum number of records, you might consider including more than three electronic databases.

Determining which databases to use requires careful deliberation and expert guidance. As is well-described at this point, each literature review and synthesis is unique; the reviewer needs to carefully explore available database options, preferably under the guidance of a medical librarian. Given the hundreds of available databases, selection may initially be a daunting task. Thus, deciding which databases house the key articles relevant to your topic is a pragmatic place to begin your database selection. A medical librarian can inform the reviewer of which databases may be useful and can facilitate finding access to using specific and/or less commonly used databases. You might initiate your search with a credible database from which you anticipate a high data yield. For example, reviewers may begin with a search of PubMed or Ovid MEDLINE. You can search the remainder of your selected electronic databases in descending order of expected yield. The reviewer may be limited by which databases are available through their institutional affiliation. Some databases are highly specialized and may be difficult to access. If there is a database pertinent to your search to which you do not have access, you might verify with your medical librarian alternative access routes and/or petition your institution to purchase access for both your and other literature reviews.

There are common databases used within each health profession discipline that is committed to publishing literature relevant to each respective profession. The reviewer should attempt to search databases specific to their professional discipline, especially if a given review focuses on a topic that is highly relevant to the field. It is also imperative that the reviewer differentiates between peer-reviewed data sources and data sources that do not necessarily undergo the peer review process or same level of rigor. Table 4.1 provides a brief list of databases that are commonly used in literature reviews, which include peer-reviewed literature.

Most literature reviews across health disciplines include a MEDLINE search, accessed through either PubMed or Ovid MEDLINE. PubMed is a freely accessible database including more than 30 million citations from the biomedical literature (www.pubmed.ncbi.nlm.nih.gov). Of note, when you access PubMed via your institution's virtual library or repository website, you will automatically be linked/have access to the journals to which your institution subscribes. If you plan to include a reproducible search strategy in a literature review publication, providing a PubMed search strategy is generally reproducible for most reviewers, because of the availability of PubMed.

Exhibit 4.5 demonstrates considerations for a reviewer determining which databases to search for when conducting a literature review and synthesis.

Other Types of Searching

Following the execution of the electronic search, you might leverage other types of literature searching including handsearching, author searching, and/or ancestry searching. **Handsearching:** With handsearching, the reviewer will typically read the reference lists of the literature or data sources that are eligible for inclusion in the review (Fink, 2020). Handsearching allows for retrieval of any eligible articles that may have been missed by the electronic database search; overlooking articles can occur even after the execution of a detailed, comprehensive electronic database search following the structuring of a search strategy. A reviewer can also handsearch the tables of contents of relevant journals (Booth et al., 2016), particularly the tables of contents in highly relevant special editions. Keep in mind that there is an association between the accuracy of handsearching results and the knowledge and expertise of the person(s) conducting the handsearch (Ganann et al., 2010). Thus, we recommend that either the person(s) conducting the handsearch be well-versed on the topic; alternatively, multiple people who are at least familiar with the topic

TABLE 4.1   HEALTHCARE LITERATURE DATABASE EXAMPLES

Database, Website, Topic Area
AMED https://health.ebsco.com/products/amed-the-allied-and-complementary-medicine-database British Library database that covers alternative therapies, allied therapies, and similar subjects.
CANCERLIT www.nlm.nih.gov/pubs/techbull/nd97/nd97_nci.html NCI database for information on cancer, including the prevention, screening, treatment, and supportive care for cancer.
CINAHL www.ebscohost.com/nursing/products/cinahl-databases/cinahl-complete Database for nursing as well as allied health professionals.
Cochrane Database of Systematic Reviews www.cochranelibrary.com/cdsr/about-cdsr Cochrane Database for Cochrane Reviews as well as protocols and other information.
DARE www.crd.york.ac.uk/crdweb/ShowRecord.asp?ID=32004000332&ID=32004000332 Database of record of INAHTA publications on health technology assessment.
Embase www.elsevier.com/solutions/embase-biomedical-research Database for biomedical research and literature.
Education Resources Information Center www.ebsco.com/products/research-databases/eric Institute of Education Sciences of the U.S. Department of Education database of education literature and resources.
Ovid HealthStar http://ospguides.ovid.com/OSPguides/hstrdb.htm National Library of Medicine's database on literature on several health areas including research, services, administration, and technology.
MEDLINE/PubMed www.nlm.nih.gov/bsd/pmresources.html MEDLINE provides biomedical literature. PubMed provides free access to many MEDLINE articles.
ProQuest Dissertations www.proquest.com/?defaultdiss=true Database for open access dissertations and theses.
ProQuest LibGuides Sociological Abstracts https://proquest.libguides.com/SocAbs Database of social work, sociology, and literature of related disciplines.
PsycInfo www.apa.org/pubs/databases/psycinfo Database for research in the behavioral and social science arenas.
Scopus www.scopus.com/home.uri Comprehensive database of research from many different fields, including science.
Web of Science https://clarivate.com/webofsciencegroup/solutions/web-of-science Curated database of publisher-independent scientific literature.

AMED, allied and complementary medicine database; DARE, database of abstracts of reviews of effects.

EXHIBIT 4.5 DETERMINING WHICH DATABASES TO SEARCH

The reviewer begins the literature search by using PubMed. The reviewer has consulted with the medical librarian and an infectious disease expert. Both provide recommendations regarding which databases to search. The reviewer works closely with them on the order in which to search and they provide guidance on where the most relevant articles might be found. The reviewer creates the list accordingly. Although they will not conduct as comprehensive a search as a reviewer might execute for a Cochrane style review (due to time and resource constraints), the reviewer still wants to be sure that they choose databases where they will find the literature that is important to the question. Therefore, in addition to PubMed she chooses these databases to search:

CINAHL
Embase
Global Health Database
ProQuest Dissertation
Cochrane Database of Systematic Reviews

---

independently may conduct the handsearch and verify concordance via comparing results. **Author searching:** If there are authors who are particularly prolific in the field or on a topic that the reviewer is studying, it is helpful to search for related data sources using the identified author's name. This may require searching in different databases including non-peer reviewed databases. Be mindful of accurate spelling and use of middle initials and alternate last names. **Ancestry searching:** Other helpful search techniques include ancestry or descendancy approaches, also known as "pearl growing" or "citation mining". Once you have determined key studies ("pearls") included in your review, you can subsequently search for the literature in which these articles are now cited. Google Scholar can be helpful with ancestry or decendancy searching, as this search engine often provides links to articles that have cited a particular article.

Utilizing these multiple approaches can potentially lead the reviewer to locate more recently published related articles that have cited a key study in a given article. In general, if a significant number of relevant references are not retrieved by the search, the reviewer might consider revising the search strategy to address potential gaps and/or inaccuracies. Careful review of these missing references will provide information about keywords or MeSH terms to add, remove, or augment, or otherwise how to adapt the strategy for greater sensitivity and specificity.

Searching the Grey Literature

Grey literature refers to material that is not commercially published and is thus not searchable solely by electronic databases (Bolderston, 2008). Whether you decide to include grey literature in your search will be contingent upon your review purpose and question. Including grey literature may decrease the publication bias and may provide more conservative treatment effects (McAuley et al., 2000). Always keep in mind, however, that different types of literature undergo varying levels of peer-review rigor; some grey literature may not be peer-reviewed at all. Therefore, a careful critical appraisal and quality assessment of data sources ultimately deemed relevant for potential inclusion in your review will be necessary, a later step in the process of conducting a literature review.

There is a myriad of grey literature sources and formats. Conference proceedings are one of the most popularly referenced types of grey literature. Conference proceedings allow the reviewer to locate state-of-the-science work that is not yet published in a peer-reviewed venue and can often be located on association websites. Theses and dissertations are often reviewed for the same reason, as this format of grey literature often contains data from studies that is likely forthcoming in the peer-reviewed literature. Other sources of information include evidence-based reports released by organizations to address diverse healthcare and social service issues, as well as policy statements and government reports. Depending on the type of your literature review, you might choose to review different websites or online information (Fink, 2020).

Several databases provide linkages to and information on grey literature—far too many than can be reasonably included in this chapter. An initial list to get you started includes: GreyNet International (www.greynet.org); the Grey Literature Report (www.greylit.org), a historical resource published by the New York Academy of Medicine (which was discontinued in 2017); and OpenGrey (www.opengrey.eu), an open access resource to grey literature centered in Europe. For a cursory, non-systematic search, a reviewer might start with an easily accessible online search engine such as Google Scholar (www.scholar.google.com), which encompasses ample literature from a variety of source types, including grey literature. Remember that in addition to grey literature, the reviewer will likely retrieve peer-reviewed publications using this database, which demands that the reviewer determine whether the retrieved data source is grey literature. As many data sources are accessible within seconds via the internet, it is incumbent upon the reviewer to carefully evaluate the quality of the resources that are searched and formally included within the literature review and synthesis.

Exhibit 4.6 details how a reviewer determines how to search the grey literature.

EXHIBIT 4.6 DETERMINING HOW TO SEARCH THE GREY LITERATURE

The reviewer wants to ensure that they locate abstracts that may have been published at global conferences on immigrant health and decides to search Google Scholar.

The reviewer reviews the World Health Organization (WHO) website, as WHO is involved in the care of diverse global populations, including persons who have immigrated.

They also review the organizational websites for the Center for Migration Studies and the International Council of Nurses to verify whether any relevant research studies may be included in the literature review.

As the reviewer conducts the search, they make a note to themselves if there are specific organizations that are mentioned frequently in the literature that they have not yet searched and reviewed these resources.

ACTIVITIES
Activity I

As a nurse or other healthcare or health policy professional, you have selected a topic that you want to explore and have carefully crafted your review question. You are now preparing to choose your search terms. Ideally, you have a medical librarian who can provide guidance during this process. You proceed with the following steps:

1. Craft your review question.
2. Choose your search terms (may be informed by a preliminary search of the literature).
3. Identify at least one to three MeSH terms that are relevant to your review.
4. Determine at least one to three text words that are relevant to your review.
5. Establish your search restrictions.

Activity II

You are a reviewer who is studying how to effectively manage chronic pain. In response to the opioid epidemic in the United States, you are examining perspectives of individuals regarding non-pharmacological approaches to chronic back pain management. In addition to searching several traditional electronic databases, you decide to explore the grey literature.

1. List three to five websites located when you used an online search engine (e.g., Google Scholar) to search: *"non-pharmacological pain management."*
2. Review and evaluate the websites that you locate.
3. Determine whether these sources are sufficiently rigorous to include in your search and provide your rationale.

SUMMARY POINTS

It is vital that reviewers invest time into considering how they are going to develop and execute the search strategy. Completing these early stages accurately and comprehensively will lessen potential frustration and unnecessary time used toward generating limited or irrelevant results. There are several steps necessary to planning and implementing a fitting search strategy that will yield results that accurately depict the state of the science.

- Developing a search strategy is a process that allows the reviewer to determine how to best search the vast array of global literature as part of conducting a literature review and synthesis. There are several steps involved in the search strategy process including determining the intent of the search, developing the literature review team, choosing the search terms, and executing the search strategy. It is important to invest time upfront to prepare for the search, thinking through the various steps involved in search strategy development and execution. Following a systematic approach will reduce the likelihood of bias and ensure comprehensive identification of all available and relevant literature. It is also useful to concretely and precisely document the search, as this information will be needed when writing up the methods of the review and ensuring replicability.

- The reviewer should be able to articulate the intent of the search by providing a clear purpose and scope of the review. A clear review question will provide guidance for determining search terms and search strategy parameters and is critical to developing an accurate search strategy.

- In addition to a medical librarian, the literature review team may potentially need at least one additional team member who has expertise specific to the review. This team member will work closely with the primary reviewer and medical librarian to determine an optimal combination of words and databases that will sensitively and specifically locate literature that is relevant to the review

- Choosing the search terms that will be used involves early exploration of search queries, using MeSH terms when possible, and use of relevant text words. It is also important to determine the search parameters.

- Executing the search strategy involves understanding the search strategy rules. Using appropriate Boolean operators, symbols, and search syntax is necessary for optimizing the search. Choosing databases carefully and following guidelines for search queries will also facilitate relevant searches. In addition to electronic database searching, reviewers might integrate supplemental forms of searching. For example, handsearching reference lists is a popular method to locate data sources that may not have been identified in the structured electronic database search. Grey literature searching can also aid in locating pertinent data sources.

We wish to thank Jennifer C. Westrick, MSLIS, AHIP, for her review and contributions to this chapter.

REFERENCES

Aromataris, E., & Riitano, D. (2014). Constructing a search strategy and searching for evidence. A guide to the literature search for a systematic review. *The American Journal of Nursing, 114*(5), 49–56. https://doi.org/10.1097/01.NAJ.0000446779.99522.f6

Boland, A., Cherry, M. G., & Dickson, R. (2017). *Doing a systematic review: A student's guide* (2nd ed.). SAGE

Bolderston, A. (2008). Writing an effective literature review. *Journal of Medical Imaging and Radiation Sciences, 39*(2), 86–92. https://doi.org/S1939-8654(08)00057-X

Booth, A., Sutton, A., & Papaioannou, D. (2016). *Systematic approaches to a successful literature review* (2nd ed.). SAGE

Britannica, The Editors of Encyclopaedia. (2021). George Boole. *Encyclopedia Britannica.* https://www.britannica.com/biography/George-Boole

Cochrane Library. (2020). *About cochrane reviews.* https://www.cochranelibrary.com/about/about-cochrane-reviews

Cooper, H., & Hedges, L. V. (2009). Research synthesis as a scientific process. In H. Cooper, L. V. Hedges, & J. C. Valentine (Eds.), *The handbook of research synthesis* (pp. 3–16). Russell Sage Foundation.

Cooper, C., Booth, A., Varley-Campbell, J., Britten, N., & Garside, R. (2018). Defining the process to literature searching in systematic reviews: A literature review of guidance and supporting studies. *BMC Medical Research Methodology, 18*(1), 85-018-0545-3. https://doi.org/10.1186/s12874-018-0545-3

Dalton, J. E., Bolen, S. D., & Mascha, E. J. (2016). Publication bias: The elephant in the review. *Anesthesia and Analgesia, 123*(4), 812–813. https://doi.org/10.1213/ANE.0000000000001596

Eden, J., Levit, L., Berg, A., Morton, S., & Committee on Standards for Systematic Reviews of Comparative Effectiveness Research, & Institute of Medicine. (Eds.) (2011). *Finding what works in health care: Standards for systematic review.* The National Academies Press.

Fink, A. (2020). *Conducting research literature reviews: From the internet to paper* (5th ed.). SAGE

Galvan, J. L., & Galvan, M. C. (2017). *Writing literature reviews: A guide for students of the social and behavioral sciences* (7th ed.). Routledge, Taylor & Francis Group.

Ganann, R., Ciliska, D., & Thomas, H. (2010). Expediting systematic reviews: Methods and implications of rapid reviews. *Implementation Science, 5*, 56-5908-5-56. https://doi.org/10.1186/1748-5908-5-56

Joanna Briggs Institute. (2020). *Home page.* http://joannabriggs.org/

Lefebvre, C., Glanville, J., Briscoe, S., Littlewood, A., Marshall, C., Metzendorf, M. I., Noel-Storr, A., Rader, T., Shokraneh, F., Thomas, J., & Wieland, L. S. (2019). Chapter 4: Searching for and selecting studies. In J. P. T. Higgins, J. Thomas, J. Chandler, M. Cumpston, T. Li, M. J. Page, & V. A. Welch (Eds.), *Cochrane handbook for systematic reviews of interventions version 6.0* (6th ed.). Cochrane Training.

Liumbruno, G. M., Velati, C., Pasqualetti, P., & Franchini, M. (2013). How to write a scientific manuscript for publication. *Blood Transfusion = Trasfusione Del Sangue, 11*(2), 217–226. https://doi.org/10.2450/2012.0247-12

McAuley, L., Pham, B., Tugwell, P., & Moher, D. (2000). Does the inclusion of grey literature influence estimates of intervention effectiveness reported in meta-analyses? *Lancet, 357*(9237), 1228–1231.

Munn, Z., Peters, M., Stern, C., Tufanaru, C., McArthur, A., & Aromataris, E. (2018). Systematic review or scoping review? Guidance for authors when choosing between a systematic or scoping review approach. *BMC Medical Research Methodology, 18*(1), 143. https://doi.org/10.1186/s12874-018-0611-x

PRISMA. (2021). *Home page.* www.prisma-statement.org

Pautasso, M. (2013). Ten simple rules for writing a literature review. *PLoS Computational Biology, 9*(7), e1003149. https://doi.org/10.1371/journal.pcbi.1003149

Whittemore, R. (2005). Combining evidence in nursing research: Methods and implications. *Nursing Research, 54*(1), 56–62. https://doi.org/00006199-200501000-00008

5

Screening, Appraising, and Extracting the Literature

Susan W. Buchholz and Kirsten A. Dickins

Screening, appraising, and extracting data within the context of a literature review require dedicated time, focus, and critical thinking.

CHAPTER OUTLINE

- Objectives
- Screening the Literature
- Critically Appraising and Assessing the Quality of the Literature
- Hierarchy of Evidence and Practice
- Data Extraction
- Using Screening and Data Extraction Software
- Using Reference Management Software
- Activities
- Summary Points
- References

At this point, you have now developed the search strategy, formally executed the search, and documented each step, including tracking all of the sources located. The next phase of the literature review and synthesis process begins with screening the literature against established eligibility criteria. Specifically, after establishing eligibility (inclusion/exclusion) criteria, you will conduct title and abstract screening, and then full-text screening, to determine which literature will be formally integrated into your review. After an eligibility determination has been made on each data source, all included literature will be critically appraised and assessed against quality standards. If the data source meets critical appraisal or quality assessment criteria, you will complete data extraction. Often, critical appraisal and quality assessment follows an established process, using software or an online platform, in addition to a reference manager.

LEARNING OBJECTIVES

In this chapter, we discuss how to screen, appraise, and extract data from the literature that will be included in your literature review and synthesis. By the end of this chapter, you will be able to:

- Describe the steps entailed in screening the literature
- Discuss how to critically appraise and assess the quality of the literature
- Understand how to rate evidence levels of data sources
- Recognize how to use data extraction tables and technologies
- Acknowledge types of software that can be used for screening and data extraction
- Identify appropriate options for reference management software

SCREENING THE LITERATURE

After you have completed a structured search, you have often retrieved an extensive amount of literature. You now need to determine which of this literature is eligible for inclusion in your literature review and synthesis, according to the eligibility criteria established in your review protocol. You will begin by first removing all of the same literature that appears more than once in your search. This often happens as the result of executing the same search strategy in multiple databases. This process of removing duplicate literature, or the same data source that appears twice in your yielded literature, is often referred to as "de-duping." Depending on how you and your review team have decided to organize your titles and abstracts, locating duplicates may be completed automatically. While some of this process may happen automatically and/or a medical librarian may help you with de-duping, it can require work on the part of the reviewer to assess which records represent duplication, or if certain records are inadvertently overlooked in the medical librarian's initial de-duping pass. Specifically, you will still need to independently verify that all duplicates have been removed, as there might be slight variation in titles or author presentation. Therefore, it may be necessary for you to check additional information in the source literature to determine whether records are in fact duplicates or similarly related, including using the Digital Object Identifier (DOI) when it is available.

Screening, appraising, and extracting data in the context of a literature review requires dedicated time, focus, and critical thinking. It is important to have established in advance who will be the primary and secondary reviewer in the screening, critical appraisal/quality assessment, and data extraction processes. The reviewers may choose to designate a third person who can provide guidance and adjudication, especially in the situation that the primary and secondary reviewer cannot reach agreement regarding including a particular data source in their review. While it may seem more efficient to complete a review with just one reviewer, the reviewer should try to avoid that scenario if possible, as this will not optimize methodological rigor and may introduce bias into the results. In addition, the reviewer may find it challenging to publish the literature review manuscript if they determine to undertake the process independently.

Beginning the screening process, the primary and secondary reviewer need to determine ahead of time how to keep track of the total number of data sources and precisely how this shifts at each stage of the screening process. Specifically, the number of data sources retrieved from each respective database will need to be recorded and reported. Additionally, the number of data sources retrieved from the grey literature, as well as with hand searching or ancestry searching, will need to be recorded and reported. There are multiple software options available for tracking the literature screening processes. Reviewers may also choose to track this process manually. If the reviewers are not mindful of documenting these numbers from the literature review, it will become increasingly complex to track and report later in the process. While using review management software is ideal, you might also use a table in a Word document or Excel spreadsheet to document the database from which data sources were retrieved (total numbers), how many duplicates were retrieved from each database, and how many data sources were included/excluded at each stage of the screening process. Once at the full-text screening stage, the reviewers need to record and report the eligibility reasons for why the data sources were excluded. Reasons are generally tagged and reported in the language of the pre-established eligibility criteria.

Title and Abstract Screening

The next step in the process is title or title/abstract screening. You may choose to exclusively title screen first and proceed to abstract screening. However, this may in part be driven by the review software that you use, as well as the review organization with which you work, if you elect to do so. If you are, for example, working with a review network, their software and formal criteria will guide the conduct of the screening process. Essentially, this process entails independently reviewing the title or title/abstract of each review and making a determination, generally based on language, whether the data source appears to meet eligibility criteria. If yes or if it is uncertain, the data source proceeds to full-text screening.

Full-Text Screening

Once you and the other reviewer(s) determine that a data source is eligible for full-text screening, you need to obtain a full-text version of that data source. This can generally be accomplished fairly quickly if you have access to a library that either subscribes to the journal that houses the article or the library is able to obtain the data source using interlibrary loan services. This process can become challenging, however, if you do not have access to this type of library service, especially as it can be cost-prohibitive for a reviewer to directly purchase all literature that is eligible for full-text review. One method of handling this is to ensure that at least one of you on the review team has access to a library that either has the articles electronically, in print, and/or can obtain articles via interlibrary loan. Otherwise, you are dependent on either locating a free source of the article or paying for the literature. Of note, it may be the case that journal author agreements place restrictions on authors regarding with whom their article(s) can be shared.

When the full-text versions of the data sources are retrieved, it is useful to have a naming convention for saving and storing each individual data source; this will help to organize the datafiles in a way that is recognized and utilized by each member of the review team. For example, the reviewers could use the last name of the first author, the year, and the full or truncated article title (e.g., last name [2021] truncated title). The reviewers also need to determine where they will store the electronic copies of the articles. The data software that are available for this purpose often have the capability to attach each article within the literature review platform for easy storage and accessing within the platform. This is efficient for the reviewers, as they can quickly locate article sources within a shared system. Alternatively, if the review team is affiliated with one organization, you might consider a virtual private network (VPN) storage system.

Dual independent assessment of each data source against eligibility criteria is a time-involved process, requiring reading through each title/abstract, and in some instances, full-text versions of each data source. This process is imperative to the rigor of the review and it is incumbent that you and other reviewer(s) allot sufficient time for each vital step of the screening process. With some data sources, the reviewer may be able to determine relatively quickly that a particular data source does not meet the eligibility criteria, often using the language in the methods section. In other cases, to determine eligibility, it is necessary to read the entire data source multiple times. If two reviewers independently determine that a data source meets eligibility criteria, it is marked for progression to the data extraction phase. If each reviewer independently determines that a data source does not meet eligibility criteria, the primary reason for exclusion (though there may be more than one reason) must be determined and documented. Remember, reasons for exclusion related to the eligibility criteria will likely be reported in the literature review manuscript. If either or both reviewers have difficulty determining eligibility and/or reaching consensus regarding whether a data source meets eligibility criteria, the decision can be adjudicated by the third independent reviewer.

Tracking the Screening Process

In the initial screening process stage, the primary reviewer and secondary reviewers will independently assess the titles or titles/abstracts against pre-established eligibility criteria (Conn & Coon Sells, 2014). Reviewers will carefully determine what must be included in a title and/or abstract in order to be deemed eligible for inclusion. For example, if the reviewer is interested in a certain age group (e.g., neonates), and the title clearly demonstrates that neonates are not part of a study population (e.g., among older adults), the data source will automatically be excluded. After each reviewer has independently screened the titles/abstracts, all data sources for which the reviewer's eligibility determinants are concordant will either be removed or will move forward to the full-text screening phase. The reviews will converse to adjudicate any existing discrepancies regarding eligibility, sometimes requiring a third reviewer if the two reviewers are unable to reach consensus. For example, if Reviewer A determined that a data source is eligible and Reviewer B determined that the same data source is ineligible, they will explain their rationale to each other. If the two reviewers are unable to agree on an eligibility determination, they may ask that a third reviewer screen the title/abstract and share a decision and rationale. If uncertainty remains after involving a third reviewer, the team can choose to move the record onto full-text screening to gather more details. For the data sources on which two to three reviewers have determined ineligibility based on titles/abstracts, this literature is excluded at this stage. All data sources that are not excluded in the title/abstract screening stage will progress next to full-text screening. This same process as employed in the title/abstract screening stage will be mirrored in the full-text screening phase, leveraging dual independent reviewers and a third reviewer to adjudicate when necessary. Always remember that numbers and reasons for inclusion/exclusion are closely tracked at each stage.

CRITICALLY APPRAISING AND ASSESSING THE QUALITY OF THE LITERATURE

After the primary and secondary reviewer(s) have determined which data sources will be included in the review and synthesis, each data source needs to be critically appraised and assessed for quality to determine whether the data source meets established quality criteria. When a reviewer is conducting a critical appraisal of a given data source, the reviewer may be verifying that the record meets certain standards that evidence rigor. Each data source needs to be appraised to determine if it is valid, reliable, and trustworthy. In this process, the reviewer is tasked with distinguishing between the quality of the study itself versus how the study is reported (Petticrew & Roberts, 2006). The number and types of criteria assessed against in a critical appraisal and quality assessment can vary by the study methodology used in the data source being evaluated.

As with independently deciding eligibility determination on which titles/abstracts and full-texts to include during the screening process, it is recommended that two reviewers independently and critically appraise and assess the content and quality of each data source (Joanna Briggs Institute, 2017; Petticrew & Roberts, 2006; Whittemore, 2005). While one reviewer can determine the quality of studies to be included, this solo process is not considered as rigorous as using two independent appraisals and assessments. Critical appraisal and quality assessment information should be carefully documented and transparently reported. If there are major disagreements between the primary and secondary reviewer regarding the quality appraisal and quality assessment outcomes, then a third reviewer can be integrated to independently appraise, assess, and then adjudicate any discrepancies.

Using Critical Appraisal Tools

Numerous tools are available to guide the reviewers in the critical appraisal and quality assessment process. Some tools are helpful in guiding appraisal of primary empirical literature, while other tools are more useful for appraising evidence-based practice and/or quality improvement literature. Some available tools are designed to critically appraise and assess the quality of literature reviews, not individual studies. Deciding which critical appraisal and quality assessment tool(s) will be used in your literature review requires both time and careful consideration of review team members. Due to the wide variety of critical appraisal and quality assessment tools available and the variance in the type of questions asked, thoroughly read about the features of at least a few different tools before deciding which one to use.

Critical appraisal questions will also be informed by the study design and employed in the study being examined. Although there is no standard list of questions that are used for all critical appraisal and quality assessments, there are noteworthy distinctions in tools designed for appraising quantitative versus qualitative studies. There are different forms used to appraise quantitative and qualitative evidence (Joanna Briggs Institute, 2021) and the questions in the critical appraisal tools should be carefully considered to assess if they are accurately and comprehensively assessing vital aspects of the data sources. For example, questions based on validity, reliability, and applicability may be asked to appraise quantitative studies (Booth et al., 2016). In contrast, questions for qualitative data sources are often based on credibility, transferability, dependability, and confirmability (Lincoln, 1985; Salmond & Porter, 2017). Regarding quantitative studies, a randomized controlled trial will require a different set of questions than quasi experimental or non-experimental studies. It is also helpful to assess the history of the tool, including how the tool was developed, by whom, and how it has been used by previous reviewers. Investing some time to read other literature reviews that have employed the tool will provide the reviewer with an exemplar for both how the tool was used and how the results of the critical appraisal were reported.

Some reviewers prefer to develop their own critical appraisal tool. While we generally advise against this option in most cases, a reviewer may decide that this is best suited to their literature review process. If you are considering developing your own tool, validity and reliability of the tool should be established. This can be a time-intensive process and often involves a statistician or methodologist to provide tailored guidance.

Several available critical appraisal and quality assessment tools are available, including those created and supported by leading literature review organizations, as well as by reviewers who have developed and validated their own tool. The multiple available checklists, guidelines, and frameworks include those used for both quantitative and qualitative studies. Table 5.1 provides an abbreviated list of examples of critical appraisal and quality assessment tools that have been widely used, highlighting the tools that are more commonly used in healthcare-related reviews. This list is intended to provide you with a sense of the importance of choosing a critical appraisal and quality assessment tool that provides a best fit to the study design of the data source being evaluated. As you scan the literature in your topic area of interest, take notes on which critical appraisal tools have been previously used in other similar literature reviews and have potential to be applied in your own literature review. If you are including several study designs or methodologies in your review, then you may consider using multiple tools, ideally that are provided by the same organization. The primary and secondary reviewer may find it time efficient to pilot the tool(s) that you have chosen for your review with a small

TABLE 5.1 EXAMPLES OF CRITICAL APPRAISAL/QUALITY ASSESSMENT TOOLS

Organization	Critical Appraisal/Quality Assessment Tools by Study Type
Amstar 2 www.bmj.com/content/358/bmj.j4008	Systematic reviews that include randomized or non-randomized studies
Centre for Evidence Based Medicine, Oxford University www.cebm.ox.ac.uk/resources/ebm-tools/critical-appraisal-tools	Diagnostics IPD review Prognosis Qualitative studies Randomized controlled trials Systematic reviews
Effective Public Health Practice Project – McMaster University https://merst.ca/ephpp	Quantitative studies
Joanna Briggs Institute, Adelaide, Australia https://jbi.global/critical-appraisal-tools	Analytical cross-sectional studies Case-control studies Case reports Case series Cohort studies Diagnostic test accuracy studies Economic evaluations Prevalence studies Qualitative research Quasi-experimental studies Randomized controlled trials Systematic reviews Text and opinion
Public Health Resource Unit, NHS, England – Critical Appraisal Skills Programme Tools https://casp-uk.net/casp-tools-checklists	Case control studies Clinical prediction rule Cohort studies Diagnostic studies Economic evaluations Qualitative research Randomized controlled trials Systematic reviews
RoB 2.0 – A revised Cochrane risk-bias tool for randomized trials https://methods.cochrane.org/bias/resources/rob-2-revised-cochrane-risk-bias-tool-randomized-trials	Cluster-randomized parallel-group trials Individually randomized cross-over trials Individually randomized parallel-group trials
Scottish Intercollegiate Guidelines Network Checklists www.sign.ac.uk/what-we-do/methodology/checklists	Case-control studies Cohort studies Diagnostic studies Economic studies Randomized controlled trials Systematic reviews and meta-analyses
USPSTF Criteria for Assessing Internal Validity of Individual Studies https://uspreventiveservicestaskforce.org/uspstf/about-uspstf/methods-and-processes/procedure-manual/procedure-manual-appendix-vi-criteria-assessing-internal-validity-individual-studies	Case-control studies Diagnostic accuracy studies RCTs and cohort studies Systematic reviews

IPD, individual participant data; RCTs, randomized controlled trials.

number of data sources, compare the results of the two independent appraisals, and together discuss rationale regarding whether this is the best tool to apply to all data sources included in the literature review.

Addressing Bias

When conducting a literature review, it is imperative to systematically identify and attempt to address biases in the included data sources. When bias is present and embedded in the results and interpretation of the literature review, it can be representative of systematic or predictable error, which can compromise the reliability and validity of the results. There are several types of bias that should be considered and recognized by asking specific questions in the appraisal and assessment process. Table 5.2 provides examples of types of biases that can occur in certain types of studies and how to evaluate for each respective bias type (Boland et al., 2017; Greenhalgh & Brown, 2017; Salmond & Porter, 2017). Additionally, it is useful to verify whether questions regarding bias are included in the selected critical appraisal/quality assessment tool. There are many established sources of information available to expand a reviewer's understanding of bias, related to risk for bias as well as strategies to address bias in literature review processes. You might read the Agency for Healthcare Research and Quality (AHRQ) "Methods Guide for Comparative Effectiveness Reviews – Assessing the Risk of Bias of Individual Studies in Systematic Reviews of Health Care Interventions" for an overview and more detailed exploration (www.ncbi.nlm.nih.gov/pubmedhealth/PMH0077771/pdf/PubMedHealth_PMH0077771.pdf).

TABLE 5.2 EXAMPLES OF TYPES OF BIAS, RISK FOR BIAS, AND QUESTIONS TO IDENTIFY BIAS

Type of Bias	Risk for Bias	Questions to Identify Bias
Attrition bias	Participants who withdrew from a study in comparison to those who remained in the study may differ in important ways that affected or influenced study outcomes.	Were reasons for loss to follow-up reported? Was intention to treat applied?
Detection bias	Participants or participant cohorts/groups experienced differences in how outcomes were assessed.	Was there blinding of the research team members who completed the assessments?
Performance bias	Participants in different study groups received unequal care and/or treatment (difference in application of treatment protocol) by research team members.	Did blinding of the participants occur? Did blinding of research team members occur?
Reporting bias	Participant outcome reporting may not be equivalent and/or complete.	Were study outcomes determined at the beginning of the study? Were all outcomes reported on?
Selection bias	Participants selected for the study were not representative of the population of interest.	Was the study sample/participants randomized? Was an appropriate method for allocation sequence used?

Using Findings From the Critical Appraisal and Quality Assessment

There is no singular recommendation or threshold to determine whether a data source should be included in a literature review based on results of the critical appraisal and quality assessment. However, as you are selecting your critical appraisal and quality assessment tool, you will see that tools typically include at minimum a brief explanation and/or a metric that indicates whether a study meets quality standards for inclusion. While some tools use summary scores, remember that score standardization across tools varies (National Institute for Health Research, 2021). As always, there are several important factors to consider, such as the idea that there is no perfect or methodologically flawless study. Reviewers are advised to establish a minimum quality threshold to determine adequacy of the article to be included, based specifically on how results or scores from critical appraisal tools will be used. Reviewers are advised to examine each item in the critical appraisal/quality assessment tool and determine which items are key to consider when determining eligibility for their particular literature review. To maintain objectivity, it is important that the reviewer generates a rationale as to which features they determined necessary for inclusion. Whatever quality threshold, score, or criteria your team determines, you will need to justify this decision in the methods section of the literature review manuscript. In addition, reviewers will likely need to explain how critical appraisal/quality assessment tool(s) were used.

HIERARCHY OF EVIDENCE AND PRACTICE

Level of evidence is another component of data sources that is integral to examine. For a clinician, level of evidence is central when considering a data source for use in clinical decision-making. To examine the level of evidence, first identify the study design or the methodological approach. Using a hierarchy of evidence to consider studies with rigorous designs and methods allows a clinician to be confident about the study findings to be used in clinical decision making (Bettany-Saltikov & McSherry, 2016). Recognizing the level of evidence of a particular data source provides the clinician with information on how to determine what the weight or the value is that they will place on particular evidence when making clinical decisions.

Given the vastness of healthcare and social science literature, it is perhaps not surprising that there are different evidence hierarchies available (Centre for Evidence-Based Medicine, 2009; Dang & Dearholt, 2017). Just as in so many stages of the literature review process, it is essential for the reviewer to allow adequate time to examine different evidence hierarchies to be considered in the literature review process. Although there are a wide variety of evidence hierarchies available, the top level of evidence generally includes systematic reviews and meta-analyses, followed by randomized controlled trials, with the lowest level of evidence generally being expert opinion.

Although it is helpful to define evidence in a logical order, it is also instructive for the reviewers to take a step back from their work to assess the relative value of sources of data that are lower on the evidence hierarchy. For example, expert opinion on an emerging topic on which little rigorous investigation has occurred may be of tremendous value, given that expert opinion may be the only existing literature at a given timepoint. Topics that are particularly challenging to study in formalized research settings also may require the reviewer to take note of expert opinions or case reports.

Clinical Application of Hierarchies of Evidence

Of particular concern is where a participant or patient's perspective fits into the hierarchy of evidence. The unique contributions, perspectives, and acceptance of healthcare recommendations by the patient can be overshadowed or minimized when using certain hierarchies of evidence. The clinician is often experientially aware that they can provide scientifically sound recommendations for a patient, based on a review of prior studies synthesized with their own expert opinion. However, if the patient's values or desires differ, the patient is early within the stages of change regarding a certain health behavior, or the patient has too many social or structural barriers to be able to follow the clinician's recommendation, then empirical science contributions may ring hollow for the patient (Prochaska et al., 2015). An understanding of statistical likelihoods of certain clinical outcomes constitutes an important part of the clinician's decision-making process in the diagnosis and management of any given condition. However, if the patient is diagnosed with a specific condition for which the likelihood is very low from a population perspective, the low likelihood may be of little consequence for the patient who has been diagnosed with a given condition. Therefore, clinicians are advised to continuously assess patient preferences, accessibility, and satisfaction when integrating hierarchies of evidence to guide their decisions.

Understanding the profound clinical value of qualitative research is of parallel importance to ensuring that the patient's perspective is factored into the clinical decision-making process. Often, hierarchies of evidence—by nature of the type of evidence that is prioritized on them as most scientifically rigorous—can inadvertently downplay the tremendous importance of the depth of experiences added by qualitative research. Considering the findings from qualitative studies and meta-syntheses can provide a richness and nuanced portrayal of a patient, family, and community's perspective, which is harder to capture and portray using quantitative methods alone.

In addition to understanding the level of evidence within a hierarchy of evidence, the reviewers should also take note of study limitations and how these limitations can influence the interpretation of findings and potential application thereof. The reviewers should also be aware of funding sources as well as potential conflicts of interest (Eden et al., 2011) that may be influential in study focus and interpretation.

The savvy reviewer will be able to distinguish between the level of evidence, the recommendation rating, and the quality of the evidence. A study may be designed as a randomized controlled trial (high standard on the hierarchy of evidence); however, due to the results of the study, guideline author groups may determine that insufficient evidence exists upon which to base a decision. A guideline author group may also

TABLE 5.3 EXAMPLES OF GRADE APPROACHES

Canadian Task Force on Preventive Health Care grades of recommendation, assessment, development and evaluation https://canadiantaskforce.ca/methods/grade	Grades of Recommendation, Assessment, Development, and Evaluation recommendations based on: ■ Target sudience: patients/public, clinicians, policy makers and quality measure developers ■ Quality of evidence: high, moderate, low, or very low ■ Strength of recommendations: strong recommendations, conditional recommendation
GRADE approach used in Cochrane Reviews https://training.cochrane.org/grade-approach	Framework to examine the certainty of the evidence in five domains: Risk of bias Inconsistency Indirectness Imprecision Publication bias
U.S. Preventive Services Task Force grade definitions https://uspreventiveservicestaskforce.org/uspstf/about-uspstf/methods-and-processes/grade-definitions#july2012	Grades with recommendations: A: Benefit is substantial: Offer or provide service B: Benefit is moderate: Offer or provide service C: Benefit is small: Make individually based decision D: No benefit or harms outweigh benefits: Discourage use of service I: Insufficient evidence available: Make individually based decision Further information is provided on high, moderate, and low levels of certainty.

determine that current evidence shows that harms associated with a certain treatment or intervention may outweigh the benefit. Table 5.3 provides examples of three GRADE approach sets to inform patient care recommendations.

DATA EXTRACTION

Data extraction is the process by which you will begin to assemble the collected data to organize, arrange, and catalogue the available evidence (Machi & McEnvoy, 2016). There are several data extraction strategies. You may choose to use a data extraction form created by your review team (home-grown data extraction forms), forms provided by your institution, or standardized forms from an external organization. It is worth noting that you may use different forms and fields for extraction for different data source types, such as quantitative versus qualitative studies (Joanna Briggs Institute, 2021). All members of your review team should be trained on how to use the data extraction forms in a standardized manner. We recommend that for your first (or second or third) review that you use an established form rather than one created by your review team; doing so will ensure that all pertinent data are collected, risk of errors in transcription are minimized, and a higher likelihood of precision and recording is achieved. Regardless of the data extraction form that your review team selects, there should be discussion of and an agreement on all fields of extraction, as well as on how the data extraction process will be undertaken.

TABLE 5.4 THE 15 "Ws" OF DATA EXTRACTION

1. **W**hat is the article identifier?	Unique identifier of the article or data source
2. **W**hat was the year of publication?	Year published
3. **W**ho wrote the article?	Authors of article or data source
4. **W**here was the article located?	Journal, website, other venue
5. **W**hat was the purpose?	Purpose of study or data source
6. **W**hat was the design?	Study design, methodology
7. **W**ho are the participants?	Sample size, participant characteristics
8. **W**here was the study conducted?	City, country, continent in which study was conducted
9. **W**hat was the intervention?	Intervention characteristics
10. **W**hat was studied?	Primary and secondary outcomes
11. **W**hat measures were used?	Description of variable measurement
12. **W**hich analytic method was used?	Analytic approach
13. **W**hat was found?	Study results
14. **W**hat framework was used?	Guiding theory or framework
15. **W**hat other fields of interest exist?	Other related areas of note

There are broad extraction categories that reviewers generally follow. Beyond those broad categories, however, data extraction sheets can include a variety of different items or categories. The level of depth required by the questions can also vary dependent on the intent or structuring of a data extraction form. Table 5.4 provides examples of common data extraction fields. In established data extraction forms, the extraction fields will be predetermined, typically dependent on the type of study methodology and the overarching purpose of the review.

While extracting data, it is important to remember that the final data synthesis is only as good as the data that was originally extracted. Reliability of extracting information from research reports and handling methodological variations will help to increase the inter-reliability throughout the data extraction process (Cooper & Hedges, 2009). If data are not extracted with focus and accuracy, interpretation and synthesis of findings may lack accuracy (Whittemore, 2005). As emphasized earlier, to enhance consistency and objectivity of the data extraction process, all reviewers who will extract data need to determine in advance the rules that will be followed to ensure that there is precision and reliability throughout the data extraction process. The review team also needs to determine how much specificity and how much depth they want in each of the extraction categories or domains that require more than a binary "yes or no" response. Without a plan, the review team may end up having to extract data twice, repeating the extraction process with greater precision the second time around.

TABLE 5.5 EXAMPLES OF LITERATURE REVIEW MANAGEMENT PLATFORMS

Platform	Website
Comprehensive meta-analysis	www.meta-analysis.com
Covidence	www.covidence.org
DistillerSR	www.evidencepartners.com/products/distillersr-systematic-review-software
EPPI reviewer	https://eppi.ioe.ac.uk/CMS/Default.aspx?alias=eppi.ioe.ac.uk/cms/er4&
SUMARI (JBI System)	www.jbisumari.org
OpenMeta (Analyst)	www.cebm.brown.edu/openmeta#
Rayyan	https://rayyan.qcri.org/welcome
RevMan (Cochrane System)	https://training.cochrane.org/online-learning/core-software-cochrane-reviews/revman

USING SCREENING AND DATA EXTRACTION SOFTWARE

There are multiple review management software options available to aid in organizing, managing, and easily sharing the screening and data extraction phases of a literature review. The features and presentation of these platforms range from relatively simple to a higher level of sophistication; all help to streamline and facilitate electronic ease of conducting these team-based review processes. As most of the software options require payment or membership in a specific organization, the reviewers may begin by determining what review software options are accessible through their institutions. If review software is not available through an affiliated institution, the reviewer might evaluate the cost of obtaining access, assess if student rates are available when applicable, and potentially build review software costs into a project budget. Table 5.5 provides a nonexhaustive list of examples of literature review management software. These software options offer a variety of different services and features relevant to the literature review process, such as screening and data extraction streamlining.

Development of Your Own Data Extraction Tool

When resources are limited, or when the reviewers do not want to use a specific software or online package, the reviewer can opt to use word processing software such as Word documents or Excel spreadsheets; however, these options may be challenging for the less experienced reviewer and can pose challenges to the organization of a team-based process. Furthermore, if a review team chooses to create their own data extraction tool, they may want to consider using a matrix or table method to collect the data. One formatting option is including the name of the data source on the furthest left column of the table and the data fields for extraction as the top row of the table. The reviewers may also choose to develop a questionnaire for data extraction and go through the data fields using one questionnaire per data source. In the event the reviewers create their own

TABLE 5.6 EXAMPLES OF REFERENCE MANAGEMENT SOFTWARE

Software	Website
EndNote	https://endnote.com/
Mendeley	https://mendeley.com
Papers	https://www.papersapp.com/
RefWorks	https://www.refworks.com/
Zotero	https://www.zotero.org/

tool, it will require time to determine what broad categories need to be covered, what specific questions need to be asked, and what are potential responses to the specified questions. When reviewers develop their own data extraction tool, we recommend piloting this data extraction tool with a small number of studies to begin testing for validity and reliability, particularly inter-rater reliability.

USING REFERENCE MANAGEMENT SOFTWARE

Most professional reviewers suggest the use of a reference management software (Lium-bruno et al., 2013) to expediently organize the many references often necessary in a thorough literature review and synthesis. Important considerations pertinent to selecting a reference manager include cost, accessibility, ease of use, functionality, and preference for or subscription to a reference manager by an affiliated institution. Once references have been added or imported into the reference management software, the references can then be efficiently exported and inserted into the manuscript. Prior to formatting the paper, a reviewer can select the citation style required by their target journal (e.g., APA 7th edition, AMA 10th edition); references will automatically be formatted in the text according to the specific citation style regulations and the reference list will populate accordingly. Although there may be some manual editing required with the reference list, the organization facilitated by reference management software will save the reviewer several valuable hours. Of note, most reference management software companies offer user tutorials, often in text and video formats, as well as instructions on how users can maximize software functionality. Table 5.6 provides a non-exhaustive list of commonly used reference management software options.

ACTIVITIES
Activity I

You and another reviewer have reviewed a list of titles/abstract and full texts to screen for study eligibility following execution of a literature search. After completing title/abstract screening, you now have a list of full texts that meet eligibility criteria. You are ready to critically appraise and assess the quality of the data sources. You and the secondary reviewer each independently appraise and assess each of the included data sources, and are coming back together to review your evaluations. Toward this end, you both go the CASP website (www.casp-uk.net/casp-tools-checklists) and choose the appropriate checklist. After each of you completes the checklists you compare notes and answer the following questions.

1. How did each of you respond to the items in the CASP checklist?
2. Were there any differences in your responses to the items in the checklist? If so, how do you plan to resolve those differences (e.g., third party adjudicator)?
3. Was there anything unexpected about the critical appraisal process that you had not anticipated? If so, how did you handle the unexpected component of the process?
4. Are you able to locate any examples of where these tools have been used in the literature? If so, how were they reported and/or used to make a decision on including or removing a data source within a literature review?

Activity II

You are one of two reviewers that are studying cardiovascular outcomes. You know that it is essential to extract data accurately and comprehensively from the included data sources. You determine ahead of time how you will extract the data regarding the primary and secondary outcomes of interest, including age, health history (including tobacco use), medication history, body mass index (or height and weight), blood pressure, and laboratory findings. What you notice is that not all studies reported the data in the same way, using dissimilar units of measurements. Discuss how you will resolve the discrepancies that you are finding during data extraction. Review guidelines of the American Heart Association (www.professional.heart.org/en/guidelines-and-statements), among other data sources relevant to your topic or question, as potential references to guide for data extraction.

SUMMARY POINTS

Once you have established your search strategy and executed the search, you are left with a generally extensive list of literature to review. To determine efficiently which data sources will be included in the final literature review and synthesis, there is a stepwise literature screening process that should be followed. Once title/abstract and full-text screening are completed, studies that meet eligibility criteria need to be critically appraised and assessed for quality. After the screening and critical appraisal/quality assessment stages are complete, your review team is poised to extract data from the included data sources.

• There are logical steps that are followed to screen the literature. After removing duplicates, the reviewer is ready to screen for eligibility. Reviewers will start first by screening the title, then the abstract (or title and abstract together). Records that have met eligibility criteria at this point will undergo full-text review.

- After reviewers have screened the full-texts that have met eligibility criteria, reviewers will need to determine if records are of sufficient quality to be included in the review. This evaluation is made via critical appraisal/quality assessment. There are several existing critical appraisal/quality assessment tools suited to varied data source methodologies.

- Reviewers can assess data sources to determine their placement on the hierarchy of evidence. Systematic reviews and meta-analyses are at the top of the evidence hierarchy, followed by randomized controlled trials, with opinion or editorial articles being typically toward the bottom of the hierarchy. In addition to the hierarchy of the evidence, clinicians may be interested in including (or not including) certain evidence for informing patient-centered diagnostic and management decisions centered on values and preferences.

- Although each step in the literature review and synthesis process is critical, the necessity of precise data extraction cannot be emphasized enough. At the point of data extraction, the reviewers determine what data they will include from the eligible data sources. Reviewers need to determine in advance specific processes for using the data extraction tool(s). This step needs to be completed accurately, as the synthesis is informed by the quality and uniformity of extracted data.

- There are multiple screening and data extraction software options, usually included within online literature review platforms. If the reviewer is working with an organization that conducts literature reviews, the software that will be used will likely be determined in advance. Other organizations have data extraction sheets that are in the public domain and delineate items and questions to address. There are times when a reviewer may opt to develop their own data extraction sheet, however, the tool should always be piloted and validated prior to formalized use in a literature review and synthesis.

- Using reference management software is key to efficiently organizing the literature review and synthesis. In addition, reference management software will help to decrease potential errors that can be caused by entering references manually. While there is often a cost associated with reference management software, the benefits of using this type of software are many, including streamlining and saving time throughout the team-based review process.

REFERENCES

Bettany-Saltikov, J., & McSherry, R. (2016). *How to do a systematic literature review in nursing: A step-by-step guide* (2nd ed.). Open University Press.

Boland, A., Cherry, M. G., & Dickson, R. (2017). *Doing a systematic review: A student's guide* (2nd ed.). Sage.

Booth, A., Sutton, A., & Papaioannou, D. (2016). *Systematic approaches to a successful literature review* (2nd ed.). Sage.

Centre for Evidence-Based Medicine. (2009). *Oxford centre for evidence-based medicine: levels of evidence.* https://www.cebm.ox.ac.uk/resources/levels-of-evidence/oxford-centre-for-evidence-based-medicine-levels-of-evidence-march-2009

Conn, V. S., & Coon Sells, T. G. (2014). Is it time to write a review article? *Western Journal of Nursing Research, 36*(4), 435–439. https://doi.org/10.1177/0193945913519060

Cooper, H., & Hedges, L. V. (2009). Research synthesis as a scientific process. In H. Cooper, L. V. Hedges, & J. C. Valentine (Eds.), *The handbook of research synthesis.* (pp. 3–16). Russell Sage Foundation.

Dang, D., & Dearholt, S. L. (2017). *Johns Hopkins nursing evidence-based practice: Models and guidelines* (3rd ed.). Sigma Theta Tau International.

Eden, J., Levit, L., Berg, A., Morton, S., & Committee on Standards for Systematic Reviews of Comparative Effectiveness Research, & Institute of Medicine. (Eds.) (2011). *Finding what works in health care: Standards for systematic review.* Washington, D.C.: The National Academies Press.

Greenhalgh, J., & Brown, T. (2017). Quality assessment: Where do I begin? In A. Boland, M. G. Cherry, & R. Dickson (Eds.), *Doing a systematic review: A student's guide* (2nd ed., pp. 107–130). Sage.

Joanna Briggs Institute. (2017). *Checklist for systematic reviews and research syntheses.* https://jbi.global/sites/default/files/2019-05/JBI_Critical_Appraisal-Checklist_for_Systematic_Reviews2017_0.pdf

Joanna Briggs Institute. (2021). *Critical appraisal tools.* https://jbi.global/critical-appraisal-tools

Lincoln, Y. S., & Guba, E. G. (1985). *Naturalistic inquiry.* Sage Publications.

Liumbruno, G. M., Velati, C., Pasqualetti, P., & Franchini, M. (2013). How to write a scientific manuscript for publication. *Blood Transfusion = Trasfusione Del Sangue, 11*(2), 217–226. https://doi.org/10.2450/2012.0247-12

Machi, L. A., & McEnvoy, B. T. (2016). *The literature review: Six steps to success* (3rd ed.). Corwin.

National Institute for Health Research. (2021). *PROSPERO, International prospective register of systematic reviews.* https://www.crd.york.ac.uk/PROSPERO/

Petticrew, M., & Roberts, H. (2006). *Systematic reviews in the social sciences: A practical guide.* Blackwell Publishing.

Prochaska, J. O., Redding, C. A., & Evers, K. E. (2015). The transtheoretical model and stages of change. In K. Glanz, B. K. Rimer, & K. Viswanath (Eds.), *Health behavior theory, research, and practice* (5th ed., pp. 125–140). Josey-Bass.

Salmond, S., & Porter, S. (2017). Critical appraisal. In C. Holly, S. Salmond, & M. Saimbert (Eds.), *Comprehensive systematic review for advanced practice nursing* (pp. 173–189). Springer.

Whittemore, R. (2005). Combining evidence in nursing research: Methods and implications. *Nursing Research, 54*(1), 56–62. https://doi.org/10.1097/00006199-200501000-00008

6

Synthesizing the Literature

Susan W. Buchholz and Kirsten A. Dickins

The synthesis process itself is a sizeable project. Like all sizeable projects, it is best undertaken one step at a time.

CHAPTER OUTLINE

- Objectives
- Begin the Synthesis Process
- Review the Protocol
- Review the Extracted Data
- Reflect on the Initial Findings
- Describe the Data Narratively
- Data Synthesis for Quantitative Reviews
- Data Synthesis for Qualitative Reviews
- Data Synthesis for Other Review Types
- Generate New Ideas
- Additional Synthesis Resources
- Activities
- Summary Points
- References

Throughout the synthesis process, the data that you have extracted from each included study will be uniquely combined through the ascertainment of patterns, directions, and themes. Beginning by revisiting the review protocol will allow you to recenter on the original synthesis plan. Then, it will be useful to reflect on the separate findings of each of the included data sources. You will then create a narrative synthesis based on your reflections of the findings—the patterns, directions, and themes that you have identified. Depending on the type of review, you will complete a quantitative and/or qualitative data synthesis. The quantitative data synthesis uses effect sizes of individual studies to develop the meta-analysis. Different methods are used to synthesize qualitative data. Optimally, the synthesis that you generate will bring to light novel interpretations and new ideas that guide clinical practice, research, and healthcare policy.

LEARNING OBJECTIVES

In this chapter, we discuss the steps that lead to the creation of a unique literature synthesis. By the end of this chapter, you will be able to:

- Explain how to begin the literature synthesis process
- Provide the rationale for revisiting the literature review protocol
- Execute a review of previously extracted data
- Formulate a foundation for the remainder of the work from the initial findings
- Integrate narrative data with tabular data
- Synthesize quantitative and/or qualitative data
- Differentiate data synthesis processes for varying literature review types
- Formulate novel interpretations and new ideas
- Recognize additional literature synthesis resources

BEGINNING THE SYNTHESIS PROCESS

This is the moment that your tremendous work to date comes to fruition in the form of the synthesis. Synthesis entails the process of reviewing and uniquely integrating the data extracted from individual studies, drawing conclusions based on similarities, differences, patterns, directions, and themes across the studies (Booth et al., 2016; Higgins et al., 2019b). Importantly, literature synthesis is a creative but methodical process involving the integration of existing ideas with new ideas, allowing the formation and development of novel perspectives on a selected topic or question (Torraco, 2016).

The synthesis process itself is a sizeable project. Like all sizeable projects, it is best undertaken one step at a time. Different processes may be utilized, to differing degrees, throughout the synthesis process. Box 6.1 provides a step-by-step guide to undertaking the synthesis process. We present this step-by-step guide as a general framework that you can use as a simplified starting point with the synthesis process. As you gain experience, or if you already are an experienced reviewer, you will likely engage in your own method to generate the synthesis.

The first step is to revisit your original review protocol. You have likely already done considerable work on the second step, as you have extracted data from different sources and combined them, although this is not actually synthesizing the results. With this step, it is important to take time to reflect on the work that you have already completed. Next, you will describe the data in a narrative format. Depending on the type of studies that you have

---

BOX 6.1   STEP-BY-STEP GUIDE TO SYNTHESIS

1. Revisit the review protocol
2. Review extracted data
3. Reflect on individual study findings
4. Describe the data narratively
5. Quantitative data synthesis review
6. Qualitative data synthesis review
7. Data synthesis with other types of reviews
8. Generate new ideas

---

used, you will undertake a quantitative and/or qualitative synthesis review. Both of these steps require considerable time and thought. They also require that, as a nurse or other healthcare professional, you present the work in a way that is accurate, interpretable, and meaningful to the reader. The final step will once again find you reflecting on the data in order to generate new ideas and contribute uniquely to the science.

REVISIT THE REVIEW PROTOCOL

As you begin the synthesis process, take time to return your attention to your original review protocol. Recall your original plan for conducting the synthesis; this synthesis plan should still be applicable, now that you have searched the literature, screened your studies against eligibility criteria, determined the quality of the studies that met the inclusion criteria, and extracted data from the studies that were determined to be of sufficient quality for review inclusion. It is expected that you will adhere to your original synthesis plan in the protocol that has already been registered. In the event that you wrote the protocol for an organization or wrote the protocol for a peer-reviewed publication, then you would have had the advantage of having experts review your work and they would have already provided the necessary questions to address concerns in your synthesis process, prior to completion of the protocol. If you did not have the opportunity to obtain a strong review of your protocol and discover that you now need to incorporate adaptations, then you will need to carefully document any changes, and be ready to provide justification on those changes. However, it is best to avoid that scenario if at all possible, as this will potentially raise serious concerns from editors and reviewers.

REVIEW EXTRACTED DATA

After you have revisited the original review protocol, an in-depth study of your data extraction tables may guide you in locating areas of concordance, discordance, and patterns across included studies. In your data extraction tables, you may have included information describing basic study characteristics, as well as different aspects of each study, including design, sample, setting, intervention (when applicable), and outcomes. You will also have information describing the findings from the study, including data, in order to calculate an effect size (Holly et al., 2017; Littell et al., 2008). In order to ensure precision in the data extraction process, reviewers may choose to develop a coding manual to guide the extraction and coding process. Data extracted will be used to complete the statistical analyses of the literature review (Holly et al., 2017).

After reviewing the data extraction tables, you may consider additional information that has not been included up to this point. There may be information regarding your review question, where additional data provide useful information for comparing and contrasting the studies. For example, you may not have assessed if a theoretical model was used, but now realize that this information in the generation of the synthesis would be helpful in understanding why the researchers hypothesized that an intervention would be effective. You may realize that including psychometrics of the measures used across studies is an important component of the synthesis. It is also possible that more detailed information about population sub-groups is value-added to your literature review question. In all of the aforementioned examples, adaptation to the original synthesis plan, while not ideal, may be necessary and will need to be documented and discussed in the methods section of the final report.

REFLECT ON THE INITIAL FINDINGS

At this stage in the review process, it is useful to pause and reflect on the findings across studies that have been included in your review. Take time to assess findings in totality rather than as individual studies, comparing and contrasting all of the studies that you have deemed eligible for inclusion. Review the source data and findings. Ask yourself what you are seeing as common themes across studies—What type of data is most predominant? How might readers of your review best make sense of these findings in aggregate? Read and thoughtfully reflect on the findings several times, assessing for the similarities and differences, patterns, and themes. You may find it useful to sketch out your thoughts in free form writing and drawing, noting and depicting patterns and outliers across studies. Organizing ideas requires deciding how to classify them and place them into categories, and how to connect them together. This classification provides a map for what you are describing and how you have decided to organize what you have found (including at what level of detail and specificity) (Hart, 2018). You will also want to discuss with your team observations they have made regarding similarities and differences across individual studies. Through having a "synthesis brainstorming" session with your review team, you may glean additional viewpoints or ways to make sense of the patterns or themes across the included studies. Hearing the perspectives of team members often facilitates broader consideration, generally informed by each team member's disciplinary approach and unique expertise. Prioritizing team discussion helps to avoid the siloed narrowness of individual thinking and provides an opportunity to see the potential of the synthesis from other important vantage points.

DESCRIBE THE DATA NARRATIVELY

The next step of the synthesis process involves generation of a narrative description. The narrative description that informs the synthesis can also be thought of as a qualitative component (Eden et al., 2011). The narrative synthesis can include both tabular and written descriptive sections. While data tables are valuable, tables alone do not comprise a synthesis (Petticrew & Roberts, 2006); rather, the written descriptive section generally is complemented by tabular data.

You will use your original data extraction tables for the tabular section of your narrative synthesis. You may choose to reorganize what is featured in the original data extraction tables. There may be several data tables, depending on how many characteristics, concepts, or outcomes you are featuring in the presentation of each included study. These tables may be very large and include quite a bit of detail. As you initially generate the data extraction tables, detail is helpful toward comprehensiveness. However, in the context of publication of your literature review, the number and size of your tables may be limited, due to table number restrictions. It is increasingly common to include larger tables as an online supplement, rather than printed directly within the main manuscript text.

The narrative synthesis provides information that extends beyond that in the tables, highlighting the qualitatively combined and summarized findings from the tables (Petticrew & Roberts, 2006). While it may seem straightforward to simply present the results directly from the table, combining the data allows for new conclusions to be drawn, considering all studies together. In the first part of the narrative synthesis, the reviewer may provide information regarding the studies that met inclusion criteria (Petticrew & Roberts, 2006). Eden et al. (2011) provide a guide to writing the narrative synthesis for a systematic review, including discussing each of the following components. The authors recommend that reviewers present characteristics (clinical and methodological), strengths and limitations, and patterns noted across included studies. The reviewer should assess for flaws in study design that could result in bias in the review. When describing the findings, relationships between study variables should be detailed, assessing for concordance and discordance. Reviewers should also report on the relevance of the study samples to the population of interest in the review, as well as the intervention aspects including cointerventions and comparisons, and which outcomes were assessed and with which measures. If conducting a review that does not include intervention studies for clinical use, then not all of this may apply, however much of it will still be important to include; for example, describing patterns noted across the studies.

QUANTITATIVE DATA SYNTHESIS REVIEW

In a systematic review, the quantitative data synthesis is a statistical method that calculates a summary statistic based on the results of a number of similar studies. Toward this end, we strongly advise consulting with an experienced statistician who can provide guidance and support in conducting the quantitative synthesis. The statistician can either be included on your review team from the outset or can be brought on as a consultant specifically for the quantitative synthesis process. This plan should be created and detailed in your protocol, prior to commencing the review. In the case that you are already familiar with evaluating effect sizes and using meta-analysis software, you may not require additional statistical support. The unit of measure in a quantitative systematic review is the individual study, not the individual participants included in each respective study. In the statistical analysis of a literature review, study findings may be reported first at the individual study level. Next, results may be pooled across studies in the form of a meta-analysis, provided that heterogeneity does not preclude aggregation across studies.

Effect Sizes

When statistically assessing within individual studies, an effect size can measure the numerical magnitude and direction of the association between two variables. Effect sizes can be shown in the original unit of measure (e.g., height in centimeters or inches), but are usually written as a standardized measure of effect. Using the standardized measure allows the reviewer to directly compare across studies in the literature review. There are many different types of standardized effect sizes. Table 6.1 presents three of the most common effect sizes, which are Cohen's *d*, Pearson's *r*, and odds ratios (Buchholz et al., 2016; Cooper, 2017; Littell et al., 2008). Commonly accepted sizes for interpretation are based on Cohen's work (Cohen, 1988). The type of effect size you choose is dependent on the type of data used in the variables under consideration.

Cohen's *d* is used when the outcome variable is continuous. Cohen's *d* is based on the standardized mean difference (SMD). This effect size is determined by dividing the mean difference of the variable of interest between two groups (e.g., treatment group outcome mean minus the control group outcome mean) by the pooled standard

TABLE 6.1 COMMON EFFECT SIZES

Type of Effect Size	When to Use	Interpretation	Example of Software
Cohen's *d*	Use to compare the difference between two means (e.g., the treatment group and control group)	Small = 0.20 Medium = 0.50 Large = 0.80	www.campbellcollaboration.org/escalc/html/EffectSizeCalculator-Home.php
Pearson's *r* index/ correlation coefficient *r*	Use to measure the association of the relationship between two continuous variables	Small = 0.10 Medium = 0.30 Large = 0.50	www.campbellcollaboration.org/escalc/html/EffectSizeCalculator-Home.php
Odds ratio	Use to measure the association between two dichotomous variables	Small = 1.5 Medium = 2.5 Large = 4.3	www.medcalc.org/calc/odds_ratio.php

deviation (SD) of the means from both groups (Littell et al., 2008). The SMD can be calculated with commonly used software such as Excel or SPSS or a web-based calculator (Holly et al., 2017). Cohen's *d* is applicable when different measures are used to assess the same construct across studies, offering a scale-free effect size (Cooper, 2017).

The correlation coefficient *r* is used to demonstrate both magnitude and direction of the comparison of two continuous variables. This effect size is also known as Pearson's *r* or Pearson product-moment correlation coefficient (Cooper, 2017; Littell et al., 2008). The correlation coefficient *r* represents a standardized measurement between two variables that are continuous and may be interpretable as is without further statistical adjustment. However, when using Pearson's *r* in a meta-analysis with values that are approaching the upper or lower limits of the correlation, the *r* score may require transformation into a Fisher's *Zr* before the scores are combined; this is because Pearson's *r* score is limited to −1 to +1 and can therefore result in a non-normal sampling distribution as the value approaches either limit. The *Zr* score has a normal distribution because this score is not bound by the numerical limitations of −1 to +1. Once the *Zr* is obtained, it can then be converted back into *r* for use in comparing effect sizes (Cooper, 2017; Holly et al., 2017; Littell et al., 2008).

The odds ratio (OR) conveys the effect size between two dichotomous variables. This effect size is based on the chance of an event occurring or not occurring in either the treatment or the control group. The odds for each group are derived by dividing the number of people who experienced a given event by the number of people who did not experience the same event. Therefore, the OR compares the treatment and control group by dividing the odds of an event happening in the treatment group by the odds of an event occurring in the control group (Holly et al., 2017; Littell et al., 2008). This effect size is different than the risks ratio (RR), that is also used as an effect size. The RR compares the risks of an event occurring in one group, to the risks of the same event occurring in another group (Littell et al., 2008). There is a comparison of the risk, but not the odds of the likelihood of an event occurring.

There are other statistical procedures and techniques for when effect size determination combines continuous and dichotomous data or extends beyond the scope of the common effect sizes presented here (Holly et al., 2017; Littell et al., 2008). As you are learning about these approaches, as with other forms of learning, we advise you to seek consult, such as with a statistician, and also to continually advance your personal and formal training.

Meta-Analysis

Meta-Analysis Process

The meta-analysis within a systematic review provides a single result that combines numeric findings from two or more studies (Fink, 2020). Numeric findings from a meta-analysis, in combination with narrative synthesis, provide guidance for nurses and other healthcare professionals to apply toward clinical practice, research, and health policy decisions. Rigorous meta-analyses are featured prominently in informing clinical care and critical public health decisions. Meta-analyses are not without limitations, however, both in methods and for appropriate interpretations of results in healthcare practice, research, and policy decision-making. Ideally, a reader should review not only the final numeric findings, but the individual study findings that inform the meta-analysis, developing one's own conclusion regarding the rigor of each individual study. However, while it is ideal for the reader to review the individual study findings, this may not always be possible due to time constraints of the reader (e.g., clinician that is seeing patients and quickly checks the results of a meta-analysis to inform clinical decision-making). Thus, it is incumbent on the reviewer to take sufficient care to critically appraise and assess the quality of the studies in the review, and accurately extract the data. While the meta-analysis is a component of the evidence informing a larger synthesis, it should be coupled with narrative interpretation, allowing for recognition of its meaningfulness within a given context, intervention, intended outcome, and/or population of interest.

Meta-analysis is the process of bringing together or pooling the quantitative results of the individual studies that you have included in your review into a single number. The meta-analysis process involves two primary steps. First, a standard effect size is determined from each individual study included in the review. Second, the individual effect sizes from each study are pooled together to create a single effect size that represents a summary of the individual study effect sizes (Petticrew & Roberts, 2006). A meta-analysis considers the weighting of results from individual studies, resulting in a weighted average from across all individual studies of the treatment effect (Eden et al., 2011). The summary number that results from combining the results of single studies is considered more statistically powerful than the quantitative results of the single studies individually (Fink, 2020).

While meta-analyses are considered among the most rigorous review forms, it is necessary to recognize when a meta-analysis is inappropriate to your review topic or question (Cooper, 2017; Higgins et al., 2019b). A meta-analysis is completed only on studies reporting quantitative results, requiring that included studies address the same construct and that the same or similar type control has been used in each of the studies (Cooper, 2017). The studies also must report sufficient outcome data, such that the reviewer can obtain effect sizes. If different measures are used to assess the study outcome, then the reviewer needs to be certain that they are statistically able to address heterogeneity (variation between studies) when comparing results of the different outcome measures. If there is too much heterogeneity and it is not possible to create a statistical summary of the results, the synthesis will be primarily narrative in nature (Petticrew & Roberts, 2006). There also must be sufficient studies published on a topic or question, such that a quantitative synthesis will add value beyond the results from the individual studies, especially in the setting of varied methodology.

There are many software options available for reviewers of varying experience levels. If you are conducting a systematic review under the direction of an organization such as Cochrane or Joanna Briggs Institute, you will likely use their meta-analysis software. If you are conducting the systematic review apart from an affiliated organization or institution, you will need to find your own meta-analysis software source. If you are

TABLE 6.2 META-ANALYSIS SOFTWARE

Type of Software	Description
Cochrane RevMan5 https://training.cochrane.org/online-learning/ core-software-cochrane-reviews/revman	RevMan is used for Cochrane reviews. RevMan5 software is freely available from Cochrane for Cochrane and non-Cochrane Reviews, as well as academic use. Registration is required.
CMA www.meta-analysis.com	CMA has a one- or two-year use fee and is designed for the quick completion of meta-analyses.
JBI SUMARI https://sumari.jbi.global	JBI SUMARI is used for Joanna Briggs Institute systematic reviews with a team management feature.
Excel Meta-Essentials www.erim.eur.nl/research-support/meta-essentials/ Meta XL Excel www.epigear.com/index_files/metaxl.html	Meta Essentials can be used with Excel and is a free meta-analysis tool. Meta XL can be used with Excel and is a free meta-analysis tool.
Metafor (R package) www.metafor-project.org/doku.php/installation	Metafor is used with R software to conduct meta-analyses. General knowledge of how to use R is required. R is a free software package.
SAS www.sas.com/en_us/industry/health-care.html	General knowledge of using SAS is required to complete a meta-analysis. SAS must be purchased.
SPSS www.ibm.com/docs/en/spss-statistics/ SaaS?topic=features-meta-analysis	General knowledge of using SPSS is required to complete a meta-analysis. SPSS must be purchased.
Stata Stata.com/features/meta-analysis	General knowledge of using Stata is required to complete a meta-analysis. Stata must be purchased.

CMA, comprehensive meta-analysis; SAS, statistical analysis software; SPSS, statistical package for the social sciences.

working with a statistician, they will likely have access to software or can advise you on which software to use for your meta-analysis. Table 6.2 briefly overviews a limited list of commonly used meta-analysis software. Typically, the different types of common statistical software used in healthcare science can also be used to complete a meta-analysis, however, this does require previous knowledge of how to use the software. There is free software that can be used to complete meta-analyses, worthy of being explored if funds are limited. If you are new to the meta-analysis, in addition to working with a statistician, it is useful to invest in reading the software user manuals and complete tutorials specific to the software that you have selected.

Figures

Figures are used to graphically convey patterns detected in the meta-analysis, commonly including forest plots and funnel plots (Figure 6.1). The forest plot is comprised of the effect sizes from each individual study along with confidence intervals. The effect

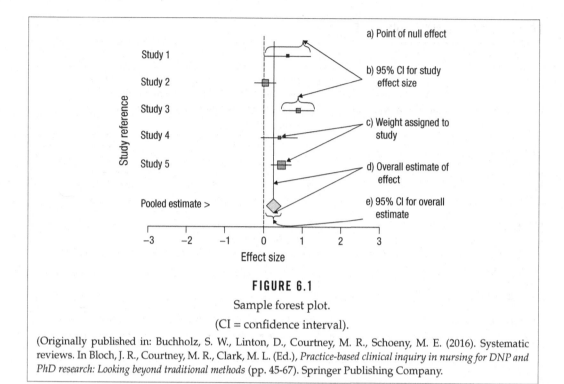

FIGURE 6.1

Sample forest plot.

(CI = confidence interval).

(Originally published in: Buchholz, S. W., Linton, D., Courtney, M. R., Schoeny, M. E. (2016). Systematic reviews. In Bloch, J. R., Courtney, M. R., Clark, M. L. (Ed.), *Practice-based clinical inquiry in nursing for DNP and PhD research: Looking beyond traditional methods* (pp. 45-67). Springer Publishing Company.

sizes and confidence intervals are plotted horizontally either side of the vertical axis, with the summary estimate included at the bottom of the forest plot. Particular symbols are used to represent the components of the forest plot. Squares represent the effect size of each individual study, with a line on either side portraying the confidence interval. The size of the square represents the weight or relative relevance of a given study within the context of the literature review. At the bottom of the forest plot, a diamond demonstrates the summary or overall effect; the center of the diamond is the pooled point estimate and the edges of the diamond represent the confidence interval. If the diamond (summary statistic representation) crosses the line of no effect (vertical axis), the results are null and favor neither the treatment nor control. However, if the diamond does not touch the line of no effect (vertical axis) and rather falls on the treatment side of the line, treatment is favored. If the diamond is positioned on the control side, the control is favored (Holly et al., 2017; Lewis & Clarke, 2001; Petticrew & Roberts, 2006). The forest plot is generally accompanied by a table that presents the variable of interest; the name of the study; and information regarding the treatment and control group results, including the sample size, effect size and confidence interval, and weight (Higgins et al., 2019b; Holly et al., 2017). Meta-analysis software can be used to create forest plots.

The funnel plot is a scatter plot that is often used in a meta-analysis to demonstrate the relationship between each individual study effect estimate against the study size or precision (Cooper, 2017; Higgins et al., 2019b; Holly et al., 2017; Petticrew & Roberts, 2006). The funnel plot (Figure 6.2) can help determine possible publication bias related

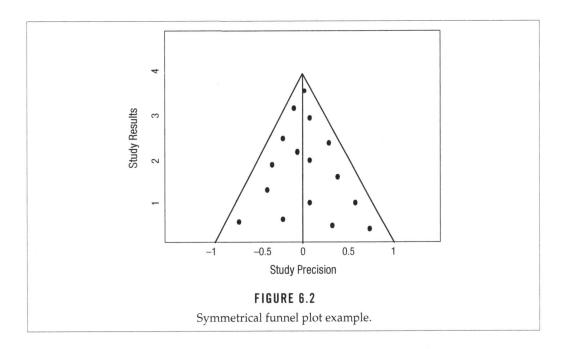

FIGURE 6.2
Symmetrical funnel plot example.

to small sample size. It is expected that larger sample sizes should produce more precise results. Typically, the effect estimates are plotted on the horizontal axis, and the standard error (standard deviation of the sample distribution) of the effect estimate is plotted on the vertical axis. Funnel plots are designed to show expected patterns, which is an inverted funnel (Cooper, 2017; Higgins et al., 2019b; Holly et al., 2017; Petticrew & Roberts, 2006). If there is funnel asymmetry and the majority of studies closer to the bottom tend to be only one side of the funnel, this raises a publication bias concern, in that smaller studies that have been conducted and do not have statistically significant results may not have been published. Similar to forest plots, meta-analysis software can be used to create the funnel plots. In the Activities section at the end of this chapter, links to articles that include forest and funnel plots are provided so that you can see visually how they are displayed.

In addition to forest plots and funnel plots, there are other figure types that can be used to convey results of meta-analyses. For example, box-and-whisker plots visually demonstrate the distribution of effect sizes (Higgins et al., 2019b). Bubble plots depict effect sizes distribution and are generally used when there is a small number of published studies (Higgins et al., 2019b). A statistician can provide additional guidance regarding the most fitting figures specific to your meta-analysis.

Vote Counting

Vote counting is a relatively straightforward method to numerically summarize the results of all individual studies. A number of different approaches can be taken toward vote counting. For example, the reviewer can tabulate results to determine if the results of each study are: (a) statistically significant in the hypothesized direction, (b) statistically significant in the direction that was not hypothesized, (c) nonsignificant (Cooper,

2017). The reviewer may choose to tally the significantly positive findings and compare those results to the number of studies with significantly negative findings (Cooper, 2017). The reviewer determines the process on counting these numbers and may for example tally these numbers or votes to determine the benefit versus harm of a treatment. Although vote counting may seem like an intuitive approach, this method can lead to incorrect conclusions as this process can be imprecise. Vote counting does not statistically account for sample size, may not include consideration of the study methods and quality of the study, and does not allow for study variable interaction in the analysis (Cooper, 2017; Higgins et al., 2019b; Petticrew & Roberts, 2006). Therefore, although there may be occasions when this method can be used, it is not advisable to do so unless you have reviewed with a statistician who is familiar with appropriate uses and strategies to address the limitations of vote counting.

Heterogeneity

Heterogeneity, or the level of variation across individual study results, is a necessary consideration in all literature reviews. Ideally, the individual studies in your literature review will demonstrate minimal heterogeneity; however, this is not always the case. The variability across studies can be either clinical, methodological, or statistical (Table 6.3; Boland et al., 2017; Eden et al., 2011; Higgins et al., 2019a; Holly et al., 2017; Petticrew & Roberts, 2006). The word *diversity* is also used to describe heterogeneity; for example, clinical diversity. To increase validity of and confidence in the results of a meta-analysis, it is vital to address all relevant types of heterogeneity observed in the studies included in your review synthesis. A reviewer can craft a narrow review question to decrease the likelihood of heterogeneity, including only a small slice of studies that are tightly relevant to a specified topic. However, this approach risks locating and including only a small number of studies. Conversely, an excessively broad review question introduces a higher likelihood of various types of heterogeneity across included studies.

When assessing for heterogeneity in a meta-analysis, the reviewer can first visually inspect the forest plot, assessing for expected overlap between confidence intervals; this step provides an initial look to grossly determine the presence of heterogeneity (Boland et al., 2017). Next, the reviewer can use a chi-square test, where a low p-value demonstrates a strong potential for heterogeneity; however, the chi-square test does

TABLE 6.3 TYPES OF HETEROGENEITY

Type of Heterogeneity	Study Component(s) That May Contribute to Heterogeneity
Clinical	Population/sample, setting, condition, intervention, outcome(s)
Methodological	Study design, risk of bias
Statistical	Random chance results, biases caused by clinical and/or methodological variability

Content adapted from Boland et al. (2017); Eden et al. (2011); Higgins et al. (2019a); Holly et al. (2017); Petticrew & Roberts (2006).

not measure the degree of heterogeneity present. This test should be used cautiously when there are only a small number of studies, as well as when small sample sizes have been used because the detection of heterogeneity in these cases is less likely. Conversely if there are many studies in the analysis, a small amount of heterogeneity may be detected, even if that heterogeneity is not clinically important (Boland et al., 2017; Higgins et al., 2019b; Holly et al., 2017). To determine the degree of heterogeneity present, the I^2 statistic must be calculated to establish a percentage of study variation attributable to heterogeneity (Boland et al., 2017; Holly et al., 2017). Caution must be used in the interpretation of the I^2 statistic, which ranges from 0% to 100%. The boundaries of the different degrees are not distinct and do have overlap. Study variation attributable to heterogeneity can be determined as not important or small (up to 40%), moderate (30%–60%), substantial (50%–90%), and considerable (75%–100%) heterogeneity (Higgins et al., 2019b).

There are various approaches to addressing heterogeneity in your literature review. The first step is verifying data accuracy through double checking numbers. In addition to double-checking data entry, check that the type of effect measure used to ensure that the correct type of effect size in concordance with the data was used in the initial analysis. Additional statistical analyses can be run, such as sub-group analyses, sensitivity analyses, and meta-regression. You may decide to report individual effect sizes and not include a meta-analysis, particularly in the setting of considerable heterogeneity, as summary analysis cannot be confidently presented. However, if you do not complete a meta-analysis, you will need to justify this decision to your audience.

Sub-group analyses can be completed when variation is found in the treatment effect to assess if different sub-groups have impacted the overall results (Littell et al., 2008; Petticrew & Roberts, 2006). These sub-group analyses should ideally be anticipated and placed in the protocol that was submitted for the literature review. Variation may lend itself to sub-group analyses to assess if there are differences between sub-groups that may not be detected through tabulating results for the whole sample or population. Variation can occur at the study design level as well as with characteristics of the population (Littell et al., 2008; Petticrew & Roberts, 2006). Variation can occur within the population of a study; for example, by gender, age, race, ethnicity, geography, and/or socioeconomic status. Variation may also be noted in study design, as well as in the type of treatments and controls. Sub-group analyses can be completed if there are different outcomes that can be divided into further categories beyond the general outcome(s) of interest. A moderator analysis can be combined with the sub-group analysis to determine the presence and impact of moderating variables that may account for a degree of difference in sub-groups outcomes (Littell et al., 2008). While sub-group analyses provide context and nuance for results, interpretation of this process must be used cautiously, because as the number of sub-group analyses increase the likelihood of a Type I error increases (a false positive, when the null hypothesis is rejected but should have been accepted) (Littell et al., 2008; Petticrew & Roberts, 2006).

Sensitivity analysis allows for the exclusion of one or multiple specific studies from the results to test whether results remain unchanged when differing assumptions are tested (Cooper, 2017; Holly et al., 2017; Littell et al., 2008; Petticrew & Roberts, 2006). Studies with differing characteristics can be excluded in each sensitivity analysis to assess for results consistency. For example, if varying study designs are used across studies, a sensitivity analysis might be used to assess only randomized controlled trials. Sensitivity analyses might be completed based on study quality, excluding studies that fall below a certain quality score to determine whether studies of lesser quality impacted the treatment effect.

Meta-regression can also be used to address concerns related to heterogeneity between sub-groups in a meta-analysis (Afari & Hung, 2018; Petticrew & Roberts, 2006). Meta-regression is a multivariable analysis that employs the multiple regression principles. In meta-regression, study characteristics that may be moderators to the treatment effect are the independent variables and the dependent variable is the effect size (Cooper, 2017; Littell et al., 2008; Petticrew & Roberts, 2006). There must be at least 10 studies for each of the moderator variables (Littell et al., 2008). With meta-regression the moderator analysis can be run simultaneously and/or sequentially (Cooper, 2017).

Missing and Limited Data

While ideal if a meta-analysis dataset does not have missing data, this is not always the case. Many types of missing data can impact the treatment effect (Cooper, 2017; Jen, 2009). Higgins et al. (2019b) note that the type of data missing includes studies, outcomes data, summary data, participants, and study-level characteristics. Specifically, if studies are missing due to an insufficient search or the results were never published, then studies may be missing. If an outcome is either selectively reported or not measured, then missing outcomes data may result. If a researcher incompletely or selectively reports results, summary data can be missing. If there is a lack of intention-to-treat analysis, as well as study attrition, then data can be missing regarding reporting on individual participants or data points in studies. If study-level characteristics are not assessed or assessed but not reported, then there is also an increase in the likelihood of missing data (Higgins et al., 2019b). The reviewer can determine how to handle missing data, such as including only available data, imputing missing data, or using statistical modeling that accounts for missing data (Higgins et al., 2019b). The reviewer may also attempt to contact the study author(s) regarding missing data. Creating a funnel plot will also help determine whether publication bias likely occurred (Cooper, 2017).

Reporting Bias

The reviewer is only able to synthesize the studies, reports, and other source documents located in the literature search process. There are multiple types of bias that may influence publication. Box 6.2 details forms of bias. It is a monumental task to search the literature extensively and comprehensively. One only has to review the search strategy of a systematic review in Cochrane or Joanna Briggs Institute to grasp the vast number

---

BOX 6.2   CONTRIBUTORS TO REPORTING BIAS

Citation bias: A review is more likely to include studies that are frequently cited, reported in high-impact journals, or are more likely to be cited due to positive treatment effects (even when low quality).

Database bias: A review is more likely to only include studies indexed in major electronic databases, thereby not including studies that meet eligibility criteria published in journals indexed in lesser accessed databases.

Funding bias: A review includes studies when results may be impacted by funding sources (e.g., pharmaceutical industry–sponsored clinical trials).

Grey literature bias: A review includes studies not published in peer-reviewed journals but rather in the grey literature, including interim findings that may not have undergone a rigorous peer-review process.

Language and country biases: A review only includes studies published in the English language or conducted in certain countries.

Multiple publication bias: A review includes multiple publications on the same study published in multiple manuscripts.

Outcome reporting bias: A review includes outcomes of studies selectively, and does not report on the outcomes as was pre-specified prior to the study starting.

Publication bias: A review is impacted by the journal editor's decision to publish studies with statistically significant results rather than non-statistically significant or null results.

Content adapted from Eden et al., 2011; Littell et al., 2008; Petticrew & Roberts, 2006.

---

of databases searched in the published literature, as well as the number of sources that are searched for the grey literature.

Reviewers should feel emboldened to include studies reporting varying results, including those that report null findings (Cooper, 2017; Petticrew & Roberts, 2006). The reviewer is always advised to thoughtfully choose a journal for submission of the review, that is preferably housed in a major database to increase accessibility of the review. Publishing all study results—including rigorously completed studies that did not demonstrate positive outcomes—is necessary in decreasing publication bias and presenting a more comprehensively accurate picture of the science (Petticrew & Roberts, 2006).

Current Cultural Changes

Culturally, increasing attention has been placed on racial, ethnic, age, and sex and gender biases as barriers to scientific funding and publication (Ginther et al., 2011, 2018). Racial, ethnic, age, and sex and gender biases have historically negatively impacted racial and gender minorities in science, technology, engineering, mathematics, and medicine (STEMM; Gosztyla et al., 2021; National Academies of Sciences, Engineering, and

Medicine, 2020). Fortunately, the tide is changing in science, including at the national level (American Association of Colleges of Nursing, 2017). The National Institutes of Health Strategic Plan 2021 to 2025 has placed a high priority on workforce diversity, including demographic diversity (National Institutes of Health, 2021). The National Academy of Science, Engineering, and Math, among other organizations, is also actively working to improve diversity, equity, and inclusion (National Academies of Sciences, Engineering, and Medicine, 2020). As more equitable societal changes occur, the scientific workforce will be more representative of the national population. From a literature synthesis perspective, this should contribute to the publication of literature reviews and syntheses completed by a more representative scientific community.

Assessing the Study Quality for Certainty of Evidence

Determining evidence certainty that is derived from a systematic review is important in guiding decision-making for nurses and other healthcare and health policy professionals. The Grading of Recommendations Assessment, Development, and Evaluation (GRADE) system, developed by the international GRADE working group, provides a method of objectively assessing the certainty of a body of evidence (Eden et al., 2011; Fink, 2020; Higgins et al., 2019b). There are eight GRADE domains used to assess for certainty of evidence. Three domains can contribute to quality rating upgrading, including: 1. large effects, 2. dose response, 3. opposing plausible residual bias and confounding. Five domains can contribute to quality rating downgrading, including: 1. risk of bias, 2. inconsistency, 3. indirectness, 4. imprecision, 5. publication bias (Eden et al., 2011). It is useful to consider these domains when synthesizing the results of your literature review. Using the GRADE profile, certainty of the evidence can be either at a very low, low, moderate, or high level. More information about GRADE can be found at the website (www.gradeworkinggroup.org).

QUALITATIVE DATA SYNTHESIS REVIEW

Qualitative data synthesis analyzes and integrates qualitative/narrative findings from across qualitative studies included in your review. Eden et al. (2011) use the term qualitative synthesis to define the section of a quantitative literature review that describes different study aspects—including study characteristics and their relationships, strengths, limitations, contributing factors to bias, and relevance of study findings. These authors also note, in contrast, that quantitative analysis refers to the meta-analysis. However, in this chapter we are using the term qualitative data synthesis to mean synthesis of qualitative data generated by a wide range of qualitative study types (Petticrew & Roberts, 2006). Qualitative methodologies used in primary studies may include phenomenology, grounded theory, ethnography, discourse analysis, feminist research, and participatory action research, content or thematic analysis, among others. Qualitative data reported in the primary studies may be generated from a variety of sources, including individual interviews, focus groups, fieldwork notes, and/or journaling (Lockwood et al., 2020). Studies in a qualitative synthesis can include one or multiple study methodologies and one or more data source types.

There are multiple distinct synthesis methods recommended by different organizations and qualitative reviewers, including but not limited to meta-aggregation, meta-synthesis, meta-ethnography, thematic analysis, narrative synthesis, grounded theory—constant comparison, narrative synthesis, meta-study, and meta-summary synthesis (Barnett-Page & Thomas, 2009; Booth et al., 2016; Centre for Reviews and Dissemination, University of York, 2009; Lockwood et al., 2020). The approach taken is driven by the question asked and methodological approach taken by the study team. The qualitative synthesis approach is also influenced by balancing between aggregation and interpretation of findings (Booth et al., 2016). Another contributing factor to the approach taken can be the type of instruction you may have received in qualitative data synthesis, as well as how team members typically conduct a qualitative data synthesis. With qualitative synthesis, rigorous methods are used for both the interpretation of qualitative studies and integrating findings within the setting of a synthesis (Fink, 2020). Following the review protocol is important in this process, adhering to your qualitative data synthesis approach plan, with appropriate adaptations.

As already noted, there is no one-size-fits-all approach to a qualitative synthesis, though there are general principles to be followed. With qualitative research, the reviewer needs to extract findings verbatim. The findings represent the authors' analytic interpretation. These findings are illustrated by participant quotations, observations from field work, or other supportive data (Lockwood et al., 2020). Qualitative data are synthesized typically using themes or constructs. Commonalities and patterns are identified across the data from each individual study (Booth et al., 2016). Different processes can be used to revisit and reflect upon the data; for example, coding for key concepts, categories, and themes. The quality of each qualitative study should also be considered when synthesizing, rating according to the level of credibility, which is unequivocal, credible, and not supported (Lockwood et al., 2020). No matter the process used, qualitative data synthesis is an iterative process and will require reading and re-reading of the studies. Steps that you have completed in the beginning of your review will be revisited as you progress in your analytic process, returning to earlier work to redefine key terms and boundaries, as well as other aspects of the synthesis (Sandelowski & Barroso, 2007).

Whichever qualitative data synthesis method you choose, we advise that you allow adequate time to extensively read and learn about the method, ideally attending a virtual or in-person training to learn from experts in your selected qualitative synthesis method. Qualitative data synthesis is complex and understanding of this type of synthesis continues to evolve. Organizations, including Cochrane and the Joanna Briggs Institute provide up-to-date resources for reviewers (Noye et al., 2011; Lockwood et al., 2020). Whichever method you choose, you will need to provide documentation and justification of the type of inquiry you have chosen, and the traditions, assumptions, and procedures associated with that inquiry (Fink, 2020). Once you are ready to write your synthesis, you can present it using a combination of different formats, including narrative, tabular, and graphical (Booth et al., 2016). When brought together, varied qualitative sources can yield new insight into a given answer or topic area, and result in a novel explanation that accounts for the findings (Booth et al., 2016). There is a new representation of understanding regarding how to interpret the original review question.

DATA SYNTHESIS WITH OTHER TYPES OF REVIEWS

In addition to the syntheses within traditional quantitative systematic reviews and myriad qualitative literature review formats, there are other types of literature review syntheses that you will either read or conduct yourself. Some of the more common literature review types that entail syntheses include text and opinion, scoping, mixed methods, and umbrella reviews. One exemplary resource for completing data synthesis with various review types can be found in the Joanna Briggs Institute Manual for Evidence Synthesis (2021).

In a text and opinion synthesis, extracted data constitute the conclusions of the author, plus text that supports the basis of these conclusions. Because the conclusions are the author's opinion, the reviewer is advised to repeatedly read the source articles to accurately comprehend the opinion being presented. As with qualitative synthesis, the conclusions of the authors need to be documented verbatim. The data synthesis is the aggregation of the findings to form a set of statements, which account for the credibility of each included source (unequivocal, credible, not supported). The findings from across sources are then synthesized into a single set of findings (McArthur et al., 2020).

The breadth and depth of scoping reviews can vary considerably. However, scoping reviews are intended to be exploratory—undertaken to generate a better understanding of a field of study, identify research gaps, assess feasibility of completing a systematic review, and provide a summary of the findings (Holly et al., 2017). Therefore, the approach to analyzing findings is to collect data and summarize the results from across source articles. Tables and figures can be used to present the results, with the main results classified under conceptual categories of particular aspects of the study design and findings (Peters et al., 2020).

Different approaches can be taken to completing a mixed-methods literature review synthesis, in which quantitative and qualitative literature are combined. Therefore, the synthesis is dependent on the type of approach chosen, which includes a convergent segregated approach (the synthesis is performed first on the quantitative, and then the qualitative data, and then integrated together), or a convergent integrated approach (synthesis occurs simultaneously with quantitative and qualitative data) (Lizarondo et al., 2020). When synthesizing data, the reviewer can either provide numerical translation for qualitative data or provide a narrative transformation of the quantitative data, or they can use a combination of these analysis types (Holly et al., 2017). Engaging in the mixed-methods synthesis review process requires an experienced literature review team.

With an umbrella review the unit that is being analyzed is not an individual study, but rather individual literature reviews. It is not recommended that you resynthesize with umbrella reviews, but instead provide a summary of the findings. Tables are used to provide an easily interpretable overview of the findings from the systematic reviews, for both quantitative and qualitative umbrella reviews. Having a strong understanding of the subject matter is needed to be able to summarize data at the level of an umbrella review (Aromataris et al., 2020; Holly et al., 2017).

GENERATE NEW IDEAS

The quantitative and qualitative synthesis that you have completed enables your capacity to summarize your findings, and importantly, generate new ideas in your own words. This process occurs through once again reflecting on what you have completed, thoughtfully considering your findings separately and in aggregate, determining what is most value added to your topic and/or field of study. We fully appreciate that clearly and accurately synthesizing information from a diverse body of literature can be challenging (Whittemore et al., 2014). While you may be able to connect the content of published articles, the emphasis is now on your own novel thoughts, conveyed to your readers in your own words—not the ideas or direct quotations of other authors.

As you reflect on your material, use the tools that make sense to you to map out what you have found and what to address next (Bolderston, 2008). When you combine content, you may realize that your ideas are not organized linearly or do not connect perfectly. You may decide to develop ideas in different areas concurrently and later reorganize them to craft a cohesive picture (Bolderston, 2008). Creating a thematic analysis of your findings provides an organizational framework for the synthesis of your findings. From your synthesis, readers should be generally aware of major achievements, main areas of contention or debate, and remaining questions in your topic area (Pautasso, 2013). Emanating from the synthesis are key implications, recommendations for clinical practice, discussion of directions and limitations for future research, and/or recommendations for health policy.

ADDITIONAL RESOURCES FOR LITERATURE SYNTHESIS

While we have provided an introductory overview of synthesis, there are multiple articles, chapters, and books that address the various processes involved in literature synthesis in great depth. We direct you to the following resources for further guidance on synthesis techniques, including meta-analysis (Box 6.3).

BOX 6.3   A STARTING LIST OF RESOURCES FOR EXPANDING YOUR LITERATURE SYNTHESIS LIBRARY

Aromataris, E., & Munn Z. (Eds.) (2020). *JBI manual for evidence synthesis.* JBI [Literature synthesis direction is available throughout the manual]. https://wiki.jbi.global/display/MANUAL/JBI+Manual+for+Evidence+Synthesis

Booth, A., Sutton, A., & Papaioannou, D. (2016). *Systematic approaches to a successful literature review* (2nd ed.). Sage. [Chapter 9: "Synthesizing and Analyzing Qualitative Studies" (pp. 215–271).]

Cooper, H. (2017). *Research synthesis and meta-analysis: A step-by-step approach* (5th ed.). Sage. [Chapter 6 "Step 5: Analyzing and Integrating the Outcomes of Studies" and Chapter 7 "Step 6: Interpreting the Evidence" (pp. 189–285).]

Eden, J., Levit, L., Berg, A., & Morton, S. (Eds.) (2011). *Finding what works in health care: Standards for systematic reviews.* The National Academies Press [Chapter 4 "Standards for Synthesizing the Body of Evidence" (pp. 155–194)]. www.ncbi.nlm.nih.gov/books /NBK209518

Holly, C., Salmond, S. W., & Saimbert, M. K. (2017). *Comprehensive systematic review for advanced practice* (2nd ed.). Springer Publishing Co. ISBN 978-0-8261-1778-6 [Multiple chapters on different types of reviews.]

Higgins, P. T., Thomas, J., Chandler, J., Cumpston, M., Li, T., Page, M. J., & Welch, V. A. (Eds.) (2019). *Cochrane handbook for systematic reviews of interventions* (2nd ed.). The Cochrane Collaboration and Wiley [Part One: Core methods (pp. 1–4310]. For the online version 6.2 2021, this section is "Part 2: Core Methods." https://training.cochrane.org/handbook /current

Littell, J. H., Corcoran, J., & Pillai, V. (2008). *Systematic reviews and meta-analysis.* Oxford University Press. [Chapter 5 "Effect Size Metrics and Pooling Methods" and "Chapter 6: addressing Bias and Variations in Effects", pp. 79–123].

ACTIVITIES
Activity I

As a pediatric healthcare professional, you are seeking evidence-based information about parenting interventions. You decide to read the systematic review and meta-analysis entitled "Parenting interventions to promote early child development in the first three years of life: A global systematic review and meta-analysis", published in 2021 by Jeong and colleagues.

www.ncbi.nlm.nih.gov/pmc/articles/PMC8109838/pdf/pmed.1003602.pdf

After you read this review article:

1. View each of the forest plots and provide an interpretation of the results in your own words.

2. Determine whether you agree with the conclusions drawn in the synthesis section of the systematic review and meta-analysis.

Activity II

As a nurse or other healthcare or health policy professional, you have been charged with advocacy for people who have a disability. You know the importance of being able to interpret scientific results for the public. You locate a review by the Campbell Collaboration, including a plain language summary. The review is titled "Multifaceted interventions for supporting community participation among adults with disabilities: A systematic review", published in 2020 by Gross and colleagues. (In this study, Hedge's g is the effect size that is used. Hedge's g is similar to Cohen's d.)

www.onlinelibrary.wiley.com/doi/epdf/10.1002/cl2.1092

www.campbellcollaboration.org/media/k2/attachments/0358_DCG_Gross_Adults_with_
disabilities_community_participation_PLS_EN.pdf

Participate in the following activities:

1. Read the systematic review and view the figures, including the funnel plot and tables with effect sizes.
2. Read the plain language summary.
3. Discuss with a colleague the results of the synthesis in this systematic review and how results were presented. What was strong about their approach? Are there areas for improvement? What would you have done similarly or differently?

SUMMARY POINTS

The literature synthesis process is the core of the literature review. It is the point at which you transform the data extracted after the literature search and bring it together to generate new understanding. Comparing and contrasting and recognizing precisely where dearth of data exists, you can meaningfully inform next research steps. The synthesized data can inform practice and policy, and guide researchers in the design and execution of future studies that advance the science.

- When beginning the literature synthesis, consider a step-by-step approach, particularly when you are new to the synthesis process.

- The first step in the synthesis process is to revisit the review protocol written prior to commencing the literature review. The data analysis and synthesis plan provides a foundation for starting your synthesis, which may be adapted.

- The next step involves revisiting the extracted data, considering the findings in totality instead of as individual studies. Compare and contrast what you know about each respective study, including the study design, participant characteristics, and main outcomes.

- After you have revisited articles, extracted the data, and before writing, truly pause and reflect on your findings. Perhaps discuss your synthesis ideas with colleagues.

- Generating the narrative synthesis is the next step. Narrative synthesis incorporates information extending beyond the tables and figures. The narrative synthesis generally aims for a rich qualitative description that is not captured with numbers alone.

- Quantitative data synthesis integrates statistical or other numerical findings of source articles. Effect sizes assess the numerical magnitude and direction of the association between two variables, and individual study effect sizes are used to create the single meta-analysis numerical finding. Forest plots provide a depiction of meta-analysis results. Heterogeneity, missing and limited data, and reporting biases, need to be addressed with quantitative data synthesis. Providing the certainty of evidence is useful in determining best evidence for practice.

- There are different approaches that can be used for qualitative data synthesis. These approaches include but are not limited to meta-aggregation, meta-synthesis, meta-ethnography, thematic analysis, narrative synthesis, grounded theory—constant comparison, narrative synthesis, meta-study, and meta-summary synthesis.

- Varied processes are followed for the analysis of text and opinion, scoping, mixed methods, and umbrella review syntheses, which are influenced by the types of source articles included.

- The generation of new ideas is the end result of an exemplary synthesis. Formulation of novel interpretations and new ideas is a result of a thoughtful synthesis approach, methodically reviewing and analyzing data, and reflecting on the findings separately and in totality.

- It is always valuable to invest in and review other synthesis sources available to guide your literature review and synthesis process. Gaining experience in receiving and integrating tangible feedback on your synthesis drafts can be equally valuable. Training coupled with direct experience will poise you to masterfully undertake and complete the synthesis process.

REFERENCES

Afari, G. K., & Hung, Y. (2018). A meta-analysis on the effectiveness of electrolyzed water treatments in reducing foodborne pathogens on different foods. *Food Control, 93*, 150–164.

American Association of Colleges of Nursing. (2017). *Diversity, equity, and inclusion in academic nursing: AACN position statement.* https://www.aacnnursing.org/News-Information/Position-Statements-White-Papers/Diversity

Aromataris, E., Fernandez, R., Godfrey, C., Holly, C., Khalil, H., & Tungpunkom, P. (2020). Chapter 10: Umbrella reviews. In E. Aromataris, & Z. Munn (Eds.), *JBI manual for evidence synthesis.* JBI. https://synthesismanual.jbi.global. https://doi.org/10.46658/JBIMES-20-11

Barnett-Page, E., & Thomas, J. (2009). Methods for the synthesis of qualitative research: A critical review. *BMC Medical Research Methodology, 9*, 59-2288-9-59. https://doi.org/10.1186/1471-2288-9-59

Boland, A., Cherry, M. G., & Dickson, R. (2017). *Doing a systematic review: A student's guide* (2nd ed.). Sage.

Bolderston, A. (2008). Writing an effective literature review. *Journal of Medical Imaging and Radiation Sciences, 39*(2), 86–92. https://doi.org/10.1016/S1939-8654(08)00057-X

Booth, A., Sutton, A., & Papaioannou, D. (2016). *Systematic approaches to a successful literature review* (2nd ed.). SAGE.

Buchholz, S. W., Linton, D., Courtney, M. R., & Schoeny, M. E. (2016). Systematic reviews. In J. R. Bloch, M. R. Courtney, & M. L. Clark (Eds.), *Practice-based clinical inquiry in nursing for DNP and PhD research: Looking beyond traditional methods* (pp. 45–67). Springer Publishing Company.

Centre for Reviews and Dissemination, University of York. (2009). *Systematic reviews: CRD's guidance for undertaking reviews in health care.* https://www.york.ac.uk/media/crd/Systematic_Reviews.pdf

Cohen, J. (1988). *Statistical power analysis for the behavioral sciences.* Lawrence, Erlbaum and Associates.

Cooper, H. (2017). *Research synthesis and meta-analysis: A step-by-step approach* (5th ed.). SAGE.

Eden, J., Levit, L., Berg, A., & Morton, S. (2011). *Finding what works in health care: Standards for systematic review.* Washington, D.C.: The National Academies Press.

Fink, A. (2020). *Conducting research literature reviews: From the internet to paper* (5th ed.). Sage.

Ginther, D. K., Basner, J., Jensen, J., Schnell, J., Kington, R., & Schaffer, W. T. (2018). Publications as predictors of racial and ethnic differences in NIH research awards. *PloS One, 11,* e0205929.

Ginther, D. K., Schaffer, W. T., Schnell, J., Masimore, B., Liu, F., Haak, L. L., & Kington, R. (2011). Race, ethnicity, and NIH research awards. *Science, 333*(6045), 1015–1019. https://doi.org/10.1126/science.1196783

Gosztyla, M. L., Kwong, L., Murray, N. A., Williams, C. E., Behnke, N., Curry, P., & Yamoah, M. (2021). Responses to 10 common criticisms of anti-racism action in STEMM. *PLoS Computational Biology, 17*(7): E1009141. https://doi.org/10.1371/journal.pcbi.1009141

Hart, C. (2018). *Doing a literature review: Releasing the research imagination* (2nd ed.). SAGE.

Higgins, J. P. T., Savović, J, Page, M. J., Elbers, R. G., Sterne, J. A. C. (2019a). Chapter 8: Assessing risk of bias in a randomized trial. In J. P. T. Higgins, J. Thomas, J. Chandler, M. Cumpston, T. Li, M. J. Page, & V. A. Welch (Eds.), *Cochrane handbook for systematic reviews of interventions version 6.0* (6th ed.). www.training.cochrane.org/handbook

Higgins, J. P. T., Thomas, J., Chandler, J., Cumpston, M., Li, T., Page, M. J., & Welch, V. A. (2019b). *Cochrane handbook for systematic reviews of interventions* (2nd ed.). Cochrane Collaboration and Wiley. www.training.cochrane.org/handbook

Holly, C., Salmond, S. W., & Saimbert, M. K. (2017). *Comprehensive systematic review for advanced practice* (2nd ed.). Springer Publishing Co.

Jen, W. (2009). Mobile healthcare services in school-based health center. *International Journal of Medical Informatics, 78*(6), 425–34.

Lewis, S., & Clarke, M. (2001). Forest plots: Trying to see the wood and the trees. *BMJ (Clinical Research Ed.), 322*(7300), 1479–1480. https://doi.org/10.1136/bmj.322.7300.1479

Littell, J. H., Corcoran, J., & Pillai, V. (2008). *Systematic reviews and meta-analysis.* Oxford University Press.

Lizarondo, L., Stern, C., Carrier, J., Godfrey, C., Rieger, K., Salmomd, S., Apostolo, J., Kirkpatrick, P., & Loveday, H. (2020). Chapter 8: Mixed methods systematic reviews. JBI. In E. Aromataris, & Z. Munn (Eds.), *JBI manual for evidence synthesis.* https://synthesismanual.jbi.global. https://doi.org/10.46658/JBIMES-20-09

Lockwood, C., Porrit, K., Munn, Z., Rittenmeyer, L., Salmond, S., Bjerrum, M., Loveday, H., Carrier, J., & Stannard, D. (2020). Chapter 2: Systematic reviews of qualitative evidence. JBI. In E. Aromataris, & Z. Munn (Eds.), *JBI manual for evidence synthesis.* https://synthesismanual.jbi.global. https://doi.org/10.46658/JBIMES-20-03

McArthur, A., Klugarova, J., Yan, H., & Florescu, S. (2020). Chapter 4. Systematic reviews of text and opinion. In E. Aromataris, & Z. Munn (Eds.), *JBI manual for evidence synthesis.* JBI. https://synthesismanual.jbi.global. https://doi.org/10.46658/JBIMES-20-05

National Academies of Sciences, Engineering, and Medicine. (2020). *Promising practices for addressing the underrepresentation of women in science, engineering, and medicine: Opening doors.* The National Academies Press. https://doi.org/10.17226/2558

National Institutes of Health. (2021). *NIH-wide strategic plan: Fiscal years 2021–2025.* https://www.nih.gov/sites/default/files/about-nih/strategic-plan-fy2021-2025-508.pdf

Noyes, J., Booth, A., Cargo, M., Flemming, K., Harden, A., Harris, J., Garside, R., Hannes, K., Pantoja, T., & Thomas, J. (2021). Chapter 21: Qualitative evidence. In J. P. T. Higgins, J. Thomas, J. Chandler, M. Cumpston, T. Li, M, J. Page, V. A. Welch (Eds.). *Cochrane handbook for systematic reviews of interventions Version 6.2 (Updated February 2021).* Cochrane. www.training.cochrane.org/handbook

Pautasso, M. (2013). Ten simple rules for writing a literature review. *PLoS Computational Biology, 9*(7), e1003149. https://doi.org/10.1371/journal.pcbi.1003149

Peters, M. D. J., Godfrey, C., McInerney, P., Munn, Z., Tricco, A. C., & Khalil, H. (2020). Chapter 11: Scoping reviews. In E. Aromataris, & Z. Munn (Eds.), *JBI manual for evidence synthesis.* JBI. https://synthesismanual.jbi.global. https://doi.org/10.46658/JBIMES-20-12

Petticrew, M., & Roberts, H. (2006). *Systematic reviews in the social sciences: A practical guide.* Blackwell Publishing.

Sandelowski, M., & Barroso, J. (2007). *Handbook for synthesizing qualitative research.* Springer.

Torraco, R. J. (2016). Writing integrative literature reviews: Using the past and present to explore the future. *Integrative Literature Review, 15*(4), 404–428. https://doi.org/10.1177/1534484316671606

Whittemore, R., Chao, A., Jang, M., Minges, K. E., & Park, C. (2014). Methods for knowledge synthesis: An overview. *Heart & Lung: The Journal of Critical Care, 43*(5), 453–461. https://doi.org/10.1016/j.hrtlng.2014.05.014

7

Publishing Your Literature Review

Susan W. Buchholz and Kirsten A. Dickins

> *When writing, recognize that creating a manuscript is an iterative process—prepare yourself and your review team to write many drafts prior to publication.*

CHAPTER OUTLINE

- Objectives
- Groundwork Activities for Writing
- Writing the Manuscript
- Options for Structuring the Synthesis
- Tips for Strengthening the Literature Review and Synthesis Manuscript
- Selecting a Target Journal
- Publication Standards
- Activities
- Summary Points
- References

You have invested valuable time and exerted exceptional effort to arrive at this point in the literature review and synthesis process. While the heavy lifting is not yet complete, you can congratulate yourself on all that you have accomplished so far. After completing the synthesis—arguably the most intellectually challenging component of the review—you are now ready to prepare to share the knowledge that you have generated. Preparing for dissemination can be arduous but is nonetheless essential to sharing your findings and making an important contribution to advancing the science. In this chapter, we provide guidance for navigating through creating the first (and subsequent) drafts of your literature review and synthesis manuscript. We also provide important information regarding submitting your manuscript to a journal or other venue for publication. There are numerous publication standards available to provide guidance on ensuring that your manuscript exemplifies the rigor needed to excel during the review process for publication.

LEARNING OBJECTIVES

In this chapter, we discuss how nurses and other healthcare professionals can compose a literature review and synthesis manuscript for publication, including tips for dissemination. By the end of this chapter, you will be able to:

- Establish authorship, including time and writing contributions expected from each author
- Describe possible methods and frameworks to guide writing a manuscript
- Determine how to best structure your literature review and synthesis manuscript
- Understand different tips for writing a manuscript
- Consider the factors pertinent to selecting a target journal
- Report on different publication standards and ideas that can be leveraged when writing a literature review

GROUNDWORK ACTIVITIES FOR WRITING

Before putting pencil to paper—or more currently relevant, fingers to keyboard—let us complete a couple of instructive groundwork activities.

Determining Authorship

We trust that by now, you have long ago established who is the primary reviewer. That reviewer is most likely the primary author; the subsequent author order, however, may differ. The primary reviewer is responsible for purposefully thinking through who has contributed to the review, in what way, and to what degree. If the contribution was substantial, then the primary reviewer might consider asking that contributor to be an author on the literature review manuscript. Once it is determined who the authors will be, the author order will need to be carefully negotiated. We recommend that you have an explicit conversation with all authors regarding expectations and determinations for author order; if this conversation has not yet transpired, there are a few guidelines that you might find helpful. The second author is often, but not always, the second reviewer in the literature review process. This person has invested considerable time and effort to usher the review to the point of manuscript publication, understands the literature that was screened and included, and knows the review manuscript in depth. Additional authors on a literature review manuscript include, for example, the medical librarian who provided expertise regarding the search strategy development and execution. Other authors may include content and/or methods experts who were purposefully included to provide specific guidance on the topic and/or approach. For instance, you may have included a statistician who contributed to a meta-analysis, or a qualitative expert who contributed to a meta-synthesis. Ultimately, it is the decision of the primary reviewer and in some instances, the mentor, to lead conversations regarding fair and ethical determination of authorship.

Time and Writing Allocation

As mentioned throughout this text, as with other aspects of the review, writing the literature review manuscript for publication requires substantial time, energy, and cognitive effort. If you are the primary reviewer, we recommend that you make certain that you have allocated adequate space and time in your schedule for writing (Bolderston, 2008). Without this protected time, it becomes difficult and arguably impossible to produce the drafts necessary to finalize and disseminate the literature review manuscript in a timely manner. The first author/primary reviewer also needs to obtain a commitment from the other authors ensuring that they will allot sufficient time to contribute to each iteration of the manuscript. The primary reviewer will also need to negotiate who will be responsible for writing and editing each respective section of the review manuscript. This typically starts with a conversation with all authors seated around the in-person or virtual table to decide who is responsible for an initial draft of each section of the manuscript and revisions thereof.

When writing, recognize that creating a manuscript is an iterative process—prepare yourself and your review team to write many drafts prior to publication. In fact, multiple drafts will likely be required as the review is shaped into a final-form manuscript ready to be submitted for review (Bolderston, 2008). The order in which the authors will review the manuscript once the initial draft is completed should be determined ahead of time. It is often most efficient for the primary author to read through the first draft; after incorporating edits, then the primary reviewer will send this draft to another author for their independent review. When the next author reviews the draft, we generally recommend using track changes, and comments for clarity for which edits were suggested by which author. After the next author has reviewed and edited the draft, then the manuscript goes to the next author for review, and so forth. The process is generally most streamlined and efficient when each author independently reviews the manuscript one person at a time—rather than sending it out to all of the authors at the same time—to avoid conflicting or opposing suggestions offered on the different manuscript versions. Managing and reconciling revisions on multiple drafts can become challenging.

It may also be useful for the authors to decide ahead of time how often they will meet to discuss the manuscript progress, for example, once weekly for 30 or 60 minutes, biweekly for 60 minutes, or another timeframe that functions optimally for the authors. We recommend regular communication without any extensive breaks, as this is essential to completing the manuscript in a timely manner. Regularly scheduled meetings should commence even if all the authors cannot be present at each meeting. Authors may also decide to have a formal written agreement on the author order, delineating who contributes to each respective section, and the time frame by which individual assignments should be completed. A formal written agreement reduces the risk for surprises and misunderstandings regarding expectations. An agreement should outline explicitly what is required from each author, what are the consequences, and the action plan in the hopefully unlikely event that an author is not able to fulfill their contribution to the commitment.

Before beginning to write the manuscript, you and the other author(s) may find it helpful to read literature reviews that are similar to your own. You have likely already located these reviews during your initial cursory review of the literature to ensure the novelty of your work. In addition to reading those reviews, locate literature reviews (which do not necessarily have to be on the same topic as yours) from the top journals that you are targeting for submission. It can be useful to see how these reviews are structured to appropriately model but not replicate in your own.

WRITING THE MANUSCRIPT

Depending on the level of authorship experience on your team, you may already have an established optimal sequence or method for writing. There are many different approaches that can be taken when writing a manuscript, and a well-developed team often already has developed a sequence of writing steps that flow well for them. If you have a method that works, we advise you to use what is effective for you and your team. Newer writers, however, may not yet have established a writing sequence. While it may seem logical to start at the introduction and write straight through to the conclusion, that may not necessarily be the most efficient or practical approach. The purpose of the review is to determine what is available in the literature pertinent to your question and to synthesize findings to generate knowledge regarding what it means for a particular clinical problem, policy issue, or population of interest.

In the event that you do not already have an effective writing method, we offer an approach to sequencing the writing of your literature review: the "Lou Fogg Method." The "Lou Fogg Method" is named after the statistician that both of the authors of this text have had the pleasure of working with on different projects (Fogg, personal communication, 2021; Wilson et al., 2018). For writing a review we recommend combining the "Lou Fogg Method" (see Box 7.1) with carefully following the Review Protocol that you worked so diligently to prepare at the beginning of your literature review and synthesis process.

Adapted "Lou Fogg Method" for Writing a Literature Review

Prior to beginning writing the manuscript, be sure to revisit your review protocol that you have been carefully following throughout the review process. If there are any

---

BOX 7.1   THE "LOU FOGG METHOD" (ADAPTED)

1. Revisit the Review Protocol
2. Center the Manuscript on the Review Purpose and Question
3. Results: Table and Figure Display of Findings
4. Results: Narrative Review of Findings
5. Methods
6. Discussion, Limitations, Implications, and Conclusion
7. Introduction
8. Abstract, Title, and Keywords

deviations that you and your review team have made, you will need to account for those in the methods of the manuscript. The next important step is to carefully revisit the review purpose and question that are at the center of your literature review and synthesis.

The next step is to display your findings. Often in literature reviews, the visual display of findings comes in the form of tables and figures. Tables and figures can include information about each included data source such as the design, sample, variables and outcomes, findings, and implications (Whittemore, 2005). Depending on the included literature, there may be considerable variance in the tables. Often, there is more than one table included to highlight different elements of the included data sources. Authors may choose to include detailed information about other aspects; for example, frameworks and theories that may have been used to guide the study, or additional information about measures used. The authors may choose to provide in-depth methodological information about each data source, including limitations. Additional tables or other graphics should include results from the synthesis; for example, a meta-analysis or thematic analysis. There is no established limit as to what the authors can and cannot include in their tables and figures, beyond the limits set by individual journals. However, at a minimum, the authors should clearly express which data sources were selected for inclusion in the review and basic information about those sources, including key findings.

In addition to a visual display of findings, the authors should provide a narrative description of the results of the synthesis. The information in the text or narrative of the literature review should complement but not duplicate what is already displayed in the tables. Writing the synthesis of findings requires considerable thought and effort. Review team members need to carefully review the findings and together determine which are most important across the included literature. How authors choose to structure this section depends on the interpretation of the findings. Typically, the authors will describe information about the individual data sources; for example, how many studies were included in the review and where the studies were conducted. All analyses used in the synthesis process should be clearly reported (Whittemore, 2005) and described in detail.

Next in the process is writing the methods section. Many decide to begin with detailing the search strategy. A description of the search and MeSH terms, keywords, and Boolean operators/combinations of terms that were used should be included. You may choose or the journal may request that you provide the detailed search strategy, often as an Appendix. Next, you will report which databases were searched and in what order. You will also note the sources of grey literature that were read and included. Eligibility criteria will be detailed to demonstrate how you determined what data sources to include versus exclude. The steps that you took to proceed through the title, abstract (or title/abstract), and full-text screening will need to be provided. Information needs to be given to note if the different stages of the title, abstract, and full-text screenings were completed independently and how disagreements between reviewers were adjudicated. The methods section should also include a description of how the literature was critically appraised.

The search and critical appraisal/quality assessment process and outcomes are generally described in either the methods or the results section of the manuscript. Due to this variance, authors should be aware if the author guidelines instruct reviewers on where to include the description of the search and critical appraisal/quality assessment. Without explicit reporting of the methods, including the search and critical appraisal/quality assessment, it is challenging for the reader to appraise the quality of the review (Cooper & Hedges, 2009; Eden et al., 2011) or the data sources within it. A flow diagram is typically used to display the results of the search strategy (PRISMA, 2021).

The discussion section typically begins with an opening paragraph that summarizes key information about the review process and outcomes, including how many data sources were ultimately included in the review. The subsequent paragraphs in the discussion provide an overview of significant review findings, in relation to what is currently known and not known on a given topic, with respect to the review purpose and question. It is important to address any potential controversies in the review, including unexpected or contradictory findings, unanswered questions, issues of potential bias, and differing opinions. It may be useful to separate the discussion into thematic areas and treat each area as its own abbreviated review and synthesis. The discussion can also be reorganized chronologically. All pertinent information from the references should be recapitulated but also synthesized by rephrasing the significance of each included data source and relating it back to the original review purpose and question.

Next, a limitations section should be included. In the limitations section, the reviewers will carefully consider restrictions of particular methods or results, noting how these restrictions may influence the findings, interpretations, or any generalizations. Moreover, the authors should detail how each respective limitation was addressed to the best of the reviewer team's ability. Some reviewers may also choose to highlight specific strengths of the review. Each section may standalone, or they may be embedded into the discussion, depending on the preferred format of the targeted journal.

Implications for research, practice, or policy, are also generally relayed within the discussion section. The implications section answers the important question of the "so what" of the review, specifically as to whether the literature review can potentially be used to inform future research, clinical practice, or health policy. The implications section can also address key findings or major points of the review for the reader, including knowledge gaps that researchers should consider exploring in the future. To answer these important implications, refer to not only the included data sources, but also to the broader literature on the topic, bringing pertinent points to the fore, and synthesizing and reflecting on pivotal issues.

The conclusion can be written after the authors have completed writing the discussion; alternatively, the authors may opt to compose the conclusion after writing the introduction. While the conclusion is short, it is an integral component of the manuscript, as it summarizes succinctly the literature review process and outcomes. In the conclusion, reviewers generally highlight the relative importance of their contribution, as well as a brief note on future research directions.

After the discussion is written, the authors can attend to the introduction. The manuscript will begin with the introduction section which should concisely summarize the topic of the review, the relevance to the reader and other stakeholders in the field, and the intent or purpose of the review (Bolderston, 2008). Literature supporting what is known regarding a topic, and moving into the gap in the literature that is being addressed in the literature review should be detailed in the introduction. Altogether, the introduction will provide a brief summary that creates a framework for the readers that guides the remainder of the paper by demonstrating relevance and providing a rationale as to why the review was conducted. The transition from the introduction to the methods should emanate directly from the review protocol in which the reviewer addresses a priori the review purpose and question toward the end of the introduction. This purpose statement might be offset into a transition paragraph between the introduction and methods, although it can be a stand-alone section apart from the introduction section.

As you near the end of writing the manuscript, three key manuscript elements remain: the title, abstract, and keywords. The abstract is critical as it may be the only manuscript component that may be available freely to most readers outside of a paid database—often the most frequently or only section of the literature review that is read in its entirety. The abstract provides a succinct summary of each of the main sections of the literature review, generally in one to two sentences per section. The abstract is written in the format that the target journal requests, with a limited word count (depending on the journal, generally around 100–300 words), either in a structured or unstructured format. The title is of equal importance, both for intriguing and engaging readers, as well as increasing the article's searchability and findability. The title should be clear, informative, contain relevant elements of the topic addressed, and indicate the type of review or method used (Derish & Annesley, 2011; Ferrari, 2015). Before determining your title, first ensure that the word combination—either exactly or in very similar language—has not already been used in another publication. Additionally, keywords should be carefully determined, ideally with the guidance of a medical librarian to ensure that relevant MeSH terms are included; keywords will help to determine how easily your literature review is searched, located, and, relatedly, cited. A clearly written title and abstract complete with optimized keywords improves the ability of readers to quickly locate the article. If readers cannot locate your work, all of the time and effort invested into developing a comprehensive literature review will not be maximized with the exposure and attention that it deserves.

OPTIONS FOR STRUCTURING THE SYNTHESIS

The structure of your synthesis is reflective of the type of synthesis completed, how you have been taught to organize the synthesis, and, potentially, publication standards. This includes the statistical work that you have done with your review, when relevant. There are multiple organizational structuring options that you can use to generate and structure your synthesis, as there is not one standardized method (Oh, 2016). Box 7.2 provides four of those approaches for consideration when writing the synthesis (Nwaubeze, 2009, as cited in Iwuchukwu, 2015).

The logical flow and structure is organized around the existing literature on the topic, starting with an introduction to the topic. A justification for the literature review

---

BOX 7.2   ORGANIZATIONAL STRUCTURING OPTIONS FOR SYNTHESIS

- Logical Flow
- Conceptual or Thematic
- Methodological
- Chronological

---

and synthesis is then provided. The findings are reviewed and included data sources can be assessed from a logical as well as a statistical perspective (Whittemore, 2005). The conceptual or thematic organizational structure includes either the main concepts or themes that were identified in the synthesis. The reviewer can choose several key concepts and provide findings related to these concepts (Torraco, 2016). The reviewer can also choose different themes and describe the findings from the primary data sources that support those themes (Whittemore, 2005). The reviewer brings coherence to how the main concepts or themes form a unified idea. With the methodological organization structure, the author groups data sources together by methodological type. This type of structure works best when addressing questions that have been answered with research studies that have leveraged at minimum two different methodological approaches. The methodologies become a focal point for the literature review. Chronological organizational structure provides a review that is organized from a temporal or historical perspective on the topic. This structure works well when the reviewer wants to provide a framework to showcase a historical timeline of the origins and development of a topic or idea (Torraco, 2016).

TIPS FOR STRENGTHENING THE LITERATURE REVIEW AND SYNTHESIS MANUSCRIPT

Writing is a skill that improves over time, necessarily entailing focused practice and iterative expert feedback. There are different strategies that reviewers can leverage when they write that will promote the writing of a stronger literature review manuscript. We call these the A to I Tips (Table 7.1).

SELECTING A TARGET JOURNAL

Selecting a target journal holds substantial implications for the reach, readership, and impact of your literature review and synthesis. Determining your target journal can occur at two points in the process of writing a literature review manuscript: (a) before the writing starts, allowing the reviewers to create an outline in accordance with a journal's author instructions, or (b) after the writing is completed, with later adjustments to the draft's final form and fit for a particular journal. The advantage of selecting a journal ahead of time is that the reviewers can tailor the structure of the manuscript specifically

TABLE 7.1 THE A TO I TIPS FOR WRITING A LITERATURE REVIEW

Tips	Integration of Tips Into the Review
A = Avoid Common Mistakes	▪ Avoid lacking a clear purpose ▪ Avoid having too narrow of a focus ▪ Avoid limiting your analysis ▪ Avoid deficient structure and explanation of studies
B = Be Your Own Voice	▪ Use quotations sparingly ▪ Paraphrase as often as possible ▪ Write to motivate the audience
C = Clarity With Writing Is Critical	▪ Clarity is of paramount importance ▪ Sequence the different sections of the manuscript in the order of presentation of concepts ▪ Organization is imperative ▪ Focus only on the data that are relevant to the purpose and review question ▪ Analyses should be evident
D = Drafts Are Helpful	▪ Expect to write several drafts of the manuscript ▪ Respond discerningly to the critique provided by reviewers
E = Etiquette Is Necessary	▪ Steer away from being overly or unjustifiably critical ▪ Stick with the facts; only cite scientific evidence ▪ Do not overreach with interpretations or conclusions ▪ Avoid unfounded assumptions about other studies
F = Future Directions Are Useful	▪ Explore trends in the area or topic that you are exploring or presenting ▪ Consider and offer suggestions for future practice and policy ▪ Contemplate and provide guidance on priorities for upcoming research priorities
G = Graphics Are Important	▪ Improve readability by using visual aids, such as self-explanatory tables, exhibits, and figures ▪ Provide graphic explanations of statistical (numeric) results ▪ Present tables for key points and critical appraisals
H = Health Outcomes Matter	▪ Emphasize outcomes that are meaningful to clinical practice and health policy ▪ Produce and provide novel perspectives from synthesized evidence
I = Integrate the Findings	▪ Only include studies that meet the eligibility criteria ▪ Compare and contrast findings across the studies ▪ Offer a balanced and fair account of the findings ▪ Integrate the data to generate new concepts, themes, and ideas

Sources: Bolderston (2008), Liumbruno et al. (2013), Pautasso (2013), Souza et al. (2010), Steward (2004), Torraco (2016).

to those journal requirements; ultimately, this approach can save time in writing sections that are either too long for word count requirements or may not be included in the final published version. However, in the competitive world of peer-reviewed journals, there is no guarantee that the manuscript will be accepted for publication in your target journal. If the manuscript is declined by your target journal, it may require considerable rewriting and reformatting to be suited for submission to an alternative journal. Of note, if you are writing a literature review for an organization that expects you to submit your review to their organization for use within their publications, the venue to which you will submit may be pre-determined. The advantage of writing the manuscript without a journal in mind (option b), is that the authors may find it easier to write to the objective of simply producing a high-quality review; this version of the review can be revised and re-formatted to meet the varied requirements of different peer-reviewed journals. However, working on revisions to fit a specific journal may require considerable time and attention to detail.

Several factors must be considered when determining the target journal to which you will submit. Box 7.3 overviews potential questions to consider in the process of selecting a target journal.

One way to begin this determination is with two to three potential journals in mind—perhaps venues that publish articles pertinent to your field or the topic addressed in your literature review and synthesis. You will also want to ensure that the journal is reputable in your field; assessing impact factor can be one method to making this determination. You might also ask yourself whether you have historically or are currently serving as a peer reviewer for this journal. If so, then it is likely a journal that aligns closely with your interests and expertise and may match with the topic of your literature review and synthesis. Next, review the website of each journal to determine whether this journal publishes literature reviews. If you are working closely with a medical librarian, this person can generally provide extensive guidance on potential journals to which you might submit your literature review and synthesis.

BOX 7.3   QUESTIONS TO CONSIDER WHEN DETERMINING THE TARGET JOURNAL

- Does the journal publish articles in the same topic area as your review?
- Is there a medical librarian with whom you can work to determine the journal to which you might submit?
- Is the journal accessible to the population of readers that would be interested in the topic and findings?
- What is the impact factor of the journal?
- Does the journal publish open access articles, and if so, what is the associated fee?
- What is the journal publication acceptance rate?
- What is the typical duration from manuscript submission, to review(s), to publication for the journal (average time from submission to publication)?
- Has the journal recently published anything similar in topic or method to your literature review?
- Is there an upcoming special edition call that might be relevant to your literature review?
- Have you ensured that you are not considering a predatory journal?

Next, consider which databases the journal uses, to ensure that the journal is accessible to the population of readers that would most likely be interested in or benefit from your literature review and synthesis. Since abstracts included on PubMed abstracts are globally available free of charge, it is helpful to see if the journal is indexed in PubMed (www. pubmed.ncbi.nlm.nih.gov). For your specific field of expertise, first consider journals that are published in databases that you regularly access. For example, if you are a nurse scientist, you might verify whether the journal is indexed in CINAHL (www.ebsco.com/products/research-databases/cinahl-complete). If you are a medical researcher, you might guarantee that the journal is indexed in PubMed (https://pubmed.ncbi.nlm.nih.gov/). If you are a social worker, then you may see if the journal is indexed in SocINDEX (www. ebsco.com/products/research-databases/socindex). If you are a health policy expert, then you may determine whether the journal is indexed in Health Policy Reference Center (www.ebsco.com/products/research-databases/health-policy-reference-center). As there are fees associated with accessing data sources in most databases, ensuring that your manuscript citation is published does not necessarily mean that readers will have quick and affordable access to your literature review. Fortunately, most journals have their publications indexed in multiple databases which might enhance access to a broader readership.

Additional considerations include journal impact factor, Digital Object identifier (DOI), and open access options. As defined by Springer Nature, "The Impact Factor is the average number of citations counted in the Impact Factor year Y for articles published in the previous two years" (Springer Nature, 2021). Many academic institutions put a fair amount of weight on the impact factor of the journals in which faculty publish. In fact, the impact factor may be considered when the faculty member is preparing for promotion. It may be helpful for you to verify your institution's promotion policies if this is a factor in your career development. Another consideration is the journal's use of a DOI (Digital Object Identifier) (DOI, 2020). The DOI is a unique combination of numbers, letters, and symbols—a permanent identifier that is unique to a given publication. DOIs are gaining in their importance for being able to easily link an author with a publication. Additionally, you might verify whether the journal offers open access publication options. While there is often a fee associated with an open access article, some journals publish a limited number of manuscripts via open access at no cost to the authors.

An additional practical consideration is the publication acceptance rate. Publishing in highly subscribed peer-reviewed journals is becoming increasingly competitive. However, this should not deter you from pursuing the highest-ranked journal that is an optimal fit for your literature review and synthesis. Recognizing a low acceptance rate should not prohibit you from submitting to a journal that you believe is a good fit for your manuscript. We recommend always aiming high for your initial submission. If your literature review manuscript is not accepted, there is some validation in knowing the success rate and relative competitiveness of publishing at a certain journal. Further, this information can help you to appropriately tailor your decision as to which journal to submit to next.

There is often variance in the duration from submission, to review, to decision by a journal's editorial office and peer-review team. There are also differences across journals with respect to the duration from e-publication ahead of print to the print publication, as well as Open Access options. If you are on a strict timeline from submission to publication (e.g., for a grant submission or a promotion), you may consider working with a journal that has a relatively quick turnaround time. Some journals are recognized for reviewing manuscripts more quickly; however, this may require a fee and does not guarantee acceptance. Always be careful of predatory journals.

Supplemental strategies include reviewing recent publications in the journal and searching for special editions. This ensures that you are not submitting a literature review that is closely related to an article that has recently been published in your target journal; under such circumstances, it is unlikely that your manuscript will be sent out for review. It is also helpful to be aware of special editions that may be relevant to your literature review. Special edition calls are generally located on journal websites and within the journal contents; a special edition editor may also invite you to submit your work. If you are reviewing a topic that you know is of interest to a journal editorial board, you might verify whether there are any planned special issues. While your manuscript will still undergo the same peer-review process, including your literature review in a special issue will place it next to others on a similar topic and increase the likelihood that readers with an interest in this specific topic will locate it.

As discussed, always be mindful of the presence of predatory journals, which can often be covert, or not obvious. If you receive an email requesting your submission to a particular journal because you are an "expert" on a particular topic or in a certain field, first verify the credibility of that source. If you do not recognize the journal name, the editor or person making the request, or the university (if one is mentioned), we recommend against following up. Be cognizant of misspellings in the request, other blatant oddities such as grammatical errors, or indications regarding the cost of submitting an article—consider these as warning signs. Many faculty automatically delete emails that they consider suspicious due to the aforementioned warning signs. However, you also do not want to overlook or disregard a legitimate request for an invited article. In that case, you will likely recognize the name of the journal and/or the name of the person issuing the request. In the case of an Open Access journal request, you can verify whether it is listed in the Directory of Open Access Journals (www.doaj.org); if it is not listed at that website, then consider that it may be a predatory or otherwise not reputable journal. Another guideline that has been developed is the Think, Check, Submit website (www.thinkchecksubmit. org). This website provides guidance on identifying trustworthy journals.

There are now a multitude of useful websites that can help guide you toward identifying a journal to submit your literature review and synthesis. One of the most popular of these websites is *JANE (Journal/Author Name Estimator)*. There are also publisher-provided websites that can help you to locate potentially well-suited journals. Table 7.2 contains an abbreviated list of free websites that can be used to identify best fit target journals to which to submit your literature review and synthesis.

Preparing the Manuscript for Review Submission

Once you have established whether reviews are considered for publication in your target journal, next thoroughly read the style guide or author instructions for each respective

TABLE 7.2 RESOURCES TO IDENTIFY A TARGET JOURNAL FOR YOUR LITERATURE REVIEW

Website	Instructions
Elsevier Journal Finder https://journalfinder.elsevier.com	Input the title and abstract of the manuscript. This will match the manuscript with Elsevier journals that are potentially suitable for submission.
JANE (Journal/Author Name Estimator) https://jane.biosemantics.org	Input the title and/or abstract of the manuscript. Select "Find Journal." JANE references PubMed to identify best journal matches for submission.
Master Journal List – Web of Science Group https://mjl.clarivate.com/home	Proceed to "Already have a manuscript." Input the title or abstract of the manuscript. This tool searches multiple indices that are hosted on Web of Science. Registering for a free account is required to use this resource.
Springer Nature Journal Suggester https://journalsuggester.springer.com#	Enter the title or a text segment of the manuscript and select a subject area. The tool searches Springer Nature and BMC publications for potentially suitable journals for submission.
Wiley Journal Finder Beta https://journalfinder.wiley.com/ search?type=match	Enter the title or abstract of the manuscript. The tool searches Wiley for journals that are most likely to be suitable for submission.

journal. The style guide/author instructions will help to create a framework or outline for preparing the literature review and synthesis in accordance with the format required by the journal. Without consulting the journal's online style guide/author instructions prior to formatting the manuscript, your submission may be returned on account of not meeting specific guidelines. A detailed online style guide/author instructions will likely outline expectations for word count, section headings, and other integral manuscript features specific to each journal (e.g., key summaries/key points, content briefly summarizing the unique contributions of the literature review). Remember two rules when preparing your manuscript for submission, as noted in Box 7.4. Always review the style guide/author instructions specific to the journal to which you will submit. It may be useful to either print or have the style guide/author instructions easily accessible on your desktop, ensuring that you mark each guideline as you become certain that it is completed.

Once you have carefully formatted the literature review and readied it for submission, be sure to set aside sufficient time for the actual online submission process. There are many steps in the online submission process; reviewers who are new to this process often benefit from having an experienced mentor guide them or at least be readily available to address real-time questions. Each journal has its own set of rules and prompts for submission which should be adhered to carefully; these prompts may include notification

---

BOX 7.4   GOLDEN RULES FOR FORMATTING THE MANUSCRIPT

1. Review the Style Guide/Author Instructions
2. When in doubt, revisit Golden Rule #1

of co-authors, ensuring there are no conflicts of interests for yourself or co-authors, and providing justification of the respective contributions of each author to the final literature review and synthesis manuscript.

The Editorial Decision

When the literature review manuscript is submitted to the target journal, the journal editor will decide whether the manuscript will undergo peer-review or receive a "desk reject" decision. The initial decision by the editor typically occurs relatively quickly. If the editor chooses to not send your literature review out for an initial peer review, they may possibly choose to provide a rationale regarding this decision (e.g., topic of the literature review is an inappropriate fit for the journal's target audience). If the editor decides to send your literature review out for peer review, this will be noted in the online submission portal generally with the language "under review." After the manuscript is read and critiqued by peer reviewers, the editor will send you a response, typically by email, indicating the consensus opinion/decision made between the editor and the peer reviewers. You may receive one of the following decisions: "accept," "accept with minor revisions," "accept with major revisions," or "reject." Some editors will note that acceptance is not guaranteed after revisions are incorporated, but will reconsider the acceptance after an additional round of peer review occurs. If the literature review has been sent out for peer review, the editor will typically include the reviewer's comments with the decision, even if the literature review has received a "reject" decision. While it is disappointing to receive a rejection, it is vital for improvements to the manuscript. Before submitting to an alternative journal, we strongly recommend that you carefully read, consider, and potentially integrate the editor's and peer reviewers' comments/feedback, all toward strengthening the quality and impact of your literature review and synthesis.

Incorporating Feedback

The process of thoughtfully incorporating feedback entails multiple purposeful steps. The first stage is incorporating co-author feedback on the initial manuscript. It is not uncommon for authors on the same review to have conflicting ideas about how to present knowledge about the literature review manuscript. The resulting discourse can be a positive exchange, as it allows each author an opportunity to reflect on why and how they wrote a section for the literature review. Each co-author needs to be given the opportunity to express their opinion on the literature review manuscript. However, in the end, it is typically the primary reviewer's responsibility to decide what will (and will not) be included in the finalized literature review manuscript. In the case of a student who is the primary reviewer, if there are differing opinions on what to include in the manuscript, the student reviewer will need to work carefully with a faculty member, ideally a mentor who has expertise and a history of publishing literature reviews. If the student and faculty member cannot reach a mutually acceptable agreement about what to include, then it can be helpful to bring in another faculty member for consultation.

The second stage of feedback incorporation occurs prior to journal submission, involving integrating feedback from colleagues who are not authors on the literature review (Pautasso, 2013). It can be helpful to have experienced colleagues review your manuscript, focusing on content rather than form. While each member of the review team must meet certain criteria to ethically be listed as authors, including a comprehensive review of the final manuscript, other subject matter experts will undoubtedly offer new perspectives and provide clarity. As these expert colleagues have not been involved in the literature review process or manuscript composition, they will often note opportunities for improvement that are not obvious to the authors who may have blind spots due to their proximity to the process and outcome.

The third stage of incorporating feedback occurs after journal submission and receiving the feedback from the editor and peer reviewers. Incorporating feedback from reviewers and the editor is not only required to resubmit the manuscript but it also will improve the literature review (Pautasso, 2013). Thus, we consider thorough and thoughtful critique provided by reviewers to be a priceless gift. It is a gift of the time of the reviewers and editors, as well as expertise dedicated toward refining your literature review to become more rigorous, impactful, and therefore publishable. Read multiple times the editor and reviewer feedback—what they have asked that you and the co-authors address before resubmitting the manuscript. Next, create a reviewer critique/author response table. One approach to responding to reviewer/editor feedback is by compiling their remarks together by sections of the literature review, allowing for grouping together critiques from different reviewers into sections of the review manuscript. In the right column, you can offer responses to each specific reviewer/ editor critique, noting changes you may have made and other pertinent information (see Table 7.3). Another approach is to categorize the comments by reviewer/editor, addressing each reviewer/editor comment before moving on to the next person's comments. For example, if there are three peer reviewers, then the table would have three (potentially four) large sections—one for each reviewer (and potentially one for the

TABLE 7.3 EXAMPLE OF RESPONSE TO REVIEWER CRITIQUE TABLE

Reviewer Critique	Author Response
General:	
Title/Abstract:	
Introduction:	
Methods:	
Results:	
Discussion:	
Conclusion:	
Tables/Figures:	
Other Notes:	

editor), with smaller sections embedded in those larger sections to address specific remarks. The editor from the journal may also provide specific instructions on creating a reviewer critique/author table, that they request to be submitted with the revised manuscript. In that case, follow those instructions closely in order to not only deliver to the editor what they have requested, but to prevent you and your team from spending extra time in creating first your own table, and then one that is designed per the editor's request.

Journals may provide a set of guidelines regarding how to respond to reviewer/editor feedback; for example, including page numbers in the author responses for easy reviewer reference. If there is a preferred response to the review format, we recommend that you strictly follow the editor's suggestions. Whatever the requirements, always maintain professional etiquette, expressing gratitude for the editor and each reviewers' time and remarks. If you are asked to revise a feature of your literature review that you feel strongly should not be altered, provide a substantive and respectful rationale as to your choice to not integrate the editor or the reviewers' recommendations. You can also consider contacting the editor for guidance, if you or the co-authors are uncertain on how to proceed with an aspect of the critique.

After the literature review has been revised in accordance with multiple layers of feedback, it should be finalized for resubmission. In the literature review manuscript version that you are revising, you will be asked to make changes, possibly using bolding, font in a color other than black, highlighting, or using track changes. You will need to provide the revisions in the requested format. If the manuscript is returned to you with second or third requests for major or minor revisions, stay encouraged as you complete another round of the aforementioned process prior to publication. Without openness to critique from colleagues and an editor and/or peer reviewers, the chances of publication in a target journal are minimized.

PUBLICATION STANDARDS

As we have thoroughly explored, there does not exist one gold standard that is used for all literature reviews (Torraco, 2016). However, there are many outstanding organizational and author recommendations that provide guidance on writing an exemplary literature review and synthesis. Literature reviews and syntheses should generally start with the creation of a review protocol that provides the purpose and rationale supporting the conduct of a review, as well as establishing the eligibility criteria and methodological approach that will be adhered to throughout the literature review process. The location of protocol registration should be reported in the literature review manuscript. Readers of the review may include healthcare personnel, policymakers, funders, and/or other stakeholders; providing these readers with transparency regarding the protocol and process is helpful in informing them of how the literature review meets appropriate criteria (Moher et al., 2015) and standards of rigor (Table 7.4).

TABLE 7.4 PUBLICATION STANDARDS

Organization/Authors	Information
Cochrane https://training.cochrane.org/handbookcurrent/chapter-iii	■ Chapter iii provides key points and additional information on reporting a literature review
CONSORT www.consort-statement.org	■ CONSORT is a widely used resource for the recommendations on reporting randomized trials ■ The CONSORT website offers a checklist (25 items) and a flow diagram to use with publications of randomized controlled trials ■ The CONSORT statement does not provide recommendations for systematic review reporting
EQUATOR Network www.equator-network.org	■ The EQUATOR website provides reporting guidelines for 11 types of publications, including systematic reviews and protocols ■ The systematic review protocol refers the reader to the PRISMA guidelines
IOM: Standards for Systematic Reviews www.nap.edu/read/13059/chapter/7	■ Chapter 5, Box 5.1 offers recommended standards for reporting systematic reviews
Joanna Briggs Institute https://wiki.jbi.global/display/MANUAL 1.5+Systematic+review+standards	■ Joanna Briggs Institute has endorsed the use of PRISMA guidelines
MOOSE https://pubmed.ncbi.nlm.nih.gov/10789670 www.elsevier.com/data/promis_misc/ISSM_ MOOSE_Checklist.pdf	■ MOOSE is a checklist that can be used for publishing meta-analyses of observational studies
PRISMA – Preferred Reporting Items for Systematic Review and Meta-Analysis www.prisma-statement.org In March 2021 – New Guidelines were printed: The PRISMA (2021) statement: an updated guideline for reporting systematic reviews www.bmj.com/content/bmj/372/bmj.n71.full.pdf	■ PRISMA checklist is a 27-item list providing standards for publication ■ PRISMA (2021) for Abstracts checklist is a 12-item list for standards of the abstract ■ PRISMA (2021) flow diagram is used for identifying the databases and registers that were used to obtain records. Then, detailing information about which records were included for review and which were excluded, for what reason, and at which stage
RAMESES www.ramesesproject.org	■ RAMESES provides publication standards for reporting on realist syntheses
SQUIRE Guidelines www.squire-statement.org/index.cfm?fuseaction=Page. ViewPage&pageId=471	■ SQUIRE Guidelines are used when a reviewer is reporting on quality improvement studies

EQUATOR, Enhancing the QUAlity and Transparency Of health Research; IOM, Institute of Medicine; MOOSE, Meta-Analyses of Observational Studies in Epidemiology.

ACTIVITIES
Activity I

Your literature review manuscript is complete, including crafting of a title and abstract and selection of keywords. You have considered potential journals to which you may submit. However, you have not yet decided on your top target journal.

a. Select a journal finder website from Table 7.2. Enter the literature review title and/ or abstract. Choose three to five journals to consider. Create a table with the potential for journals with columns for: Journal, Audience, Impact Factor, Organizational Alignment (if relevant), and other information relevant for you and your review team.

b. Choose the journal that ranks at the top of the list across criteria. Revisit Table 7.4 to answer the questions. After making relevant considerations, note if answers will reinforce or weaken the likelihood of you submitting your manuscript to the selected target journal(s).

c. Meet with your co-author(s) to discuss your considerations after reviewing different journals, attempting to narrow on one target journal for potential submission. Note if the co-author(s) agree or dissent on the selected target journal.

Activity II

With your reviewing and writing experience in mind, you know that it is essential for authors of literature reviews to follow publishing standards. You decide to read an article about screen-based media use and academic performance in children and adolescents.

Citation: Adelantado-Renau, M., Moliner-Urdiales, D., Cavero-Redondo, I., Beltran-Valls, M. R., Martínez-Vizcaíno, V., & Álvarez-Bueno, C. (2019). Association between screen media use and academic performance among children and adolescents: A systematic review and meta-analysis. *JAMA Pediatrics*, *173*(11), 1058–1067. https://doi.org/10.1001/jamapediatrics.2019.3176. Epub ahead of print. PMID: 31545344; PMCID: PMC6764013.

www.ncbi.nlm.nih.gov/pmc/articles/PMC6764013/?report=printable#poi190061r19

At the beginning of the methods section, the authors note the following. "This systematic review and meta-analysis was conducted according to the Preferred Reporting Items for Systematic Reviews and Meta-Analyses (PRISMA) and the Cochrane handbook."

a. Review the PRISMA guidelines and/or Cochrane guidelines.

b. Determine whether this literature review adhered to the PRISMA and/or Cochrane guidelines. If yes, in what ways? If no, what were the main points of non-adherence?

c. Consider how the PRISMA and/or Cochrane guidelines will impact your own literature review and synthesis manuscript decisions.

SUMMARY POINTS

Describing your literature review and synthesis process and outcomes into one concise manuscript requires considerable time and cognitive commitment from you and your co-author(s). The writing and publication process is often among the most challenging for many thought leaders, including nurses and other healthcare and health policy professionals. We have provided information to streamline and simplify your writing, submission, and publication processes.

- The primary (or first) reviewer typically is the first author on the manuscript. The order for the other author(s), as well as establishment of who is writing each manuscript section, should be determined prior to beginning manuscript writing. The review team should be able to commit to regular meetings to discuss the manuscript and actively contribute to manuscript composition.

- Authors may prefer different methodological or strategic approaches to manuscript writing. Some authors already have time-tested processes that have successfully served them. If that is the case, we recommend that they continue with their established processes for writing a manuscript. However, for other reviewers who may not have that advantage, we offer an order that has worked well for us and other authors: the "Lou Fogg Method." In addition, we provide specific guidance on crafting each respective section of the literature review and synthesis manuscript.

- A sophisticated synthesis is central to a successfully published literature review. There are multiple options for formatting a synthesis, including using a logical flow, conceptual and thematic, methodological, or chronological organizational structure(s).

- There are several easily avoidable mistakes, as well as several accessible tips for strengthening a literature review and synthesis manuscript. Using your own voice, writing with clarity, being prepared to write multiple drafts, using tables and figures, and masterfully synthesizing the findings are all successful, value-added strategies. Additionally, offering recommended future direction, including for healthcare research, practice, and policy, will contribute to a stronger literature review manuscript.

- Choosing the appropriate journal for submission is important for several reasons, including a greater likelihood of being reviewed by and published in the selected target journal. There are several tools available to aid in identifying potential target journals. Moreover, there are multiple factors to consider when choosing a journal, including whether it is a reputable, peer-reviewed journal with a high impact factor. There are also predatory journals that should be noted and avoided.

- Publication standards are available to guide the writing of the literature review and synthesis manuscript. Frequently used publication standards include PRISMA, Cochrane, and EQUATOR.

REFERENCES

Bolderston, A. (2008). Writing an effective literature review. *Journal of Medical Imaging and Radiation Sciences*, *39*(2), 86–92. https://doi.org/S1939-8654(08)00057-X

Cooper, H., & Hedges, L. V. (2009). Research synthesis as a scientific process. In H. Cooper, L. V. Hedges, & J. C. Valentine (Eds.), *The handbook of research synthesis* (pp. 3–16). Russell Sage Foundation.

Derish, P. A., & Annesley, T. M. (2011). How to write a rave review. *Clinical Chemistry*, *57*(3), 388–391. https://doi.org/10.1373/clinchem.2010.160622

DOI. (2020). *The DOI system*. https://www.doi.org/

Eden, J., Levit, L., Berg, A., Morton, S., & Committee on Standards for Systematic Reviews of Comparative Effectiveness Research, & Institute of Medicine. (Eds.) (2011). *Finding what works in health care: Standards for systematic review*. The National Academies Press.

Ferrari, R. (2015). Writing narrative style literature reviews. *Medical Writing*, *24*(4), 230–235. https://doi.org/10.1179/2047480615Z.000000000329

Iwuchukwu, M. O. (2015). Literature review and use of Benjamin Bloom's taxonomy 1. *International Journal of Humanities and Cultural Studies*, *2*(3), 436–444.

Liumbruno, G. M., Velati, C., Pasqualetti, P., & Franchini, M. (2013). How to write a scientific manuscript for publication. *Blood Transfusion = Trasfusione Del Sangue*, *11*(2), 217–226. https://doi.org/10.2450/2012.0247-12

Moher, D., Shamseer, L., Clarke, M., Ghersi, D., Liberati, A., Petticrew, M., Shekelle, P., Steward, L. A., & PRISMA-P Group. (2015). Preferred reporting items for systematic review and meta-analysis protocols (PRISMA-P) 2015 statement. *Systematic Reviews*, *4*, 1-4053-4-1. https://doi.org/10.1186/2046-4053-4-1

Oh, E. G. (2016). Synthesizing quantitative evidence for evidence-based nursing: Systematic review. *Asian Nursing Research*, *10*(2), 89–93. https://doi.org/10.1016/j.anr.2016.05.001

Pautasso, M. (2013). Ten simple rules for writing a literature review. *PLoS Computational Biology*, *9*(7), e1003149. https://doi.org/10.1371/journal.pcbi.1003149

PRISMA. (2021). *PRISMA flow diagram*. http://www.prisma-statement.org/PRISMAStatement/FlowDiagram

Souza, M. T., Silva, M. D., & Carvalho, R. (2010). Integrative review: What is it? How to do it? *Einstein (Sao Paulo, Brazil)*, *8*(1), 102–106. https://doi.org/10.1590/S1679-45082010RW1134

Springer Nature. (2021). *Journal metrics*. https://www.springer.com/gp/authors-editors/journal-author/journal-author-helpdesk/impact-factor/18684

Steward, B. (2004). Writing a literature review. *British Journal of Occupational Therapy*, *67*, 495–500. https://doi.org/10.1177/030802260406701105

Torraco, R. J. (2016). Writing integrative literature reviews: using the past and present to explore the future. *Integrative Literature Review*, *15*(4), 404–428. https://doi.org/10.1177/1534484316671606

Wilson, C., Berton, E., Farnsworth, M., Fogg, L., & Bathje, M. (2018). Poster presentation "Recipe for Research." (2018), *Illinois Occupational Therapy Association Annual Conference*, Lisle, IL.

Whittemore, R. (2005). Combining evidence in nursing research: Methods and implications. *Nursing Research*, *54*(1), 56–62. https://doi.org/00006199-200501000-00008

Literature Review and Synthesis Implications on Healthcare Research, Practice, Policy, and Public Messaging

Susan W. Buchholz and Kirsten A. Dickins

Literature reviews and syntheses invaluably contribute to understanding the state-of-the-science for healthcare research, clinical practice, health policy, and public messaging.

CHAPTER OUTLINE

- Objectives
- The Multidisciplinary Value of Literature Review and Synthesis
- Implications of Literature Review and Synthesis on Healthcare Research
- Implications of Literature Review and Synthesis on Clinical Practice
- Implications of Literature Review and Synthesis on Health Policy
- Implications of Literature Review and Synthesis on Public Messaging
- Global Trends Impacting Literature Reviews and Syntheses
- Final Thoughts
- Activities
- Summary Points
- References

In this final chapter, we provide an overview of the multidisciplinary value of literature reviews and syntheses. Literature reviews and syntheses uniquely inform healthcare research, clinical practice, health policy, and media messaging for experts and the lay public. Literature reviews and syntheses can guide new understandings of the current literature and provide direction for future research. Additionally, they contribute to the knowledge databases and guidelines that clinicians use to inform practice decisions. Literature reviews and syntheses are also leveraged to accurately integrate existing information to inform relevant health policy decisions. There are different public venues that can be used to convey important knowledge gleaned from the work. Global trends continue to shape review processes and scale of impact. Once you have learned how to conduct a literature review and synthesis, you have gained a skill set that will undoubtedly serve you throughout your career.

LEARNING OBJECTIVES

In this chapter we discuss why literature reviews and syntheses are valuable across professional disciplines. By the end of this chapter, you will be able to:

- Describe how conducting a literature review and synthesis adds value across disciplines

- Understand the implications of literature review and synthesis on understanding and guiding future healthcare research endeavors

- Recognize the impact of literature review and synthesis on clinical practice decision-making

- Identify the influence of literature review and synthesis on health policy decision processes

- Determine opportunities and best practices for using literature reviews and synthesis in public messaging efforts

- Appraise global trends that influence literature review and synthesis guidelines and standards

- Summarize the integral components of the literature review and synthesis process and outcomes

THE MULTIDISCIPLINARY VALUE OF LITERATURE REVIEW AND SYNTHESIS

The existential question may occur to the reviewer sometime during the literature review and synthesis process: "Why does this matter?" Or "Why am I doing all of this work?" "Towards what end?" After all, a literature review and synthesis does require a great deal of time, focus, and energy. We would like to assure you of the host of varied reasons substantiating the value of the literature review and synthesis. One of the most obvious is the academic assignment—or that which is required of a student for a course that is part of an educational or training program. However, there is still an overarching objective informing the literature review assignment: Although it is a time-intensive endeavor for a student, it generally requires an investment of time and energy on behalf of the faculty member who is guiding the student, as well (particularly for the novice student reviewer). Literature reviews and syntheses invaluably contribute to understanding the state-of-the-science for healthcare research, clinical practice, health policy, and public messaging. Rigorously conducted literature reviews can be a powerful source of information for other researchers, regardless of the discipline. Literature reviews and syntheses provide researchers with the opportunity to see the state-of-the-science from an elevated and consolidated vantage point, making apparent where the gaps in the literature exist and providing the platform for determining focus. The reviewer and reader can become familiar not only with the precise topic being explored, but who the experts are on a given topic, popular methods employed, important findings, and recommended directions for future healthcare research. It is also possible that the reviewer may already be considered a topic expert and may even review their own work. With the knowledge gained from the literature review and synthesis process, a reviewer can decide to take their work in a variety of directions, now immersed in and informed by the literature regarding a question or topic.

There are nearly 8 billion people in the world (U.S. Census Bureau, 2021) and, throughout the world, there are healthcare scientists who diligently work to improve the health and healthcare for the citizens of individual countries and the global community. Every day, nurses and other healthcare professionals contribute knowledge to the global literature database, reporting on their studies and other scientific work. These studies are conducted and reported with respect to what is meaningful and useful for specific groups of people, accounting for cultural considerations and using this information to improve healthcare across settings (Oh, 2016). Internationally, many people have access to healthcare literature from varied resources, while significant issues persist with respect to equitable access to electronic databases and other relevant resources. Developing a diverse review team on which at least one team member has data access is one method to addressing this concern, albeit an imperfect one. Once nurses and other healthcare professionals distill resources that are most rigorous and reputable, there still remains an abundance of healthcare literature. There are multiple databases in multiple languages that house this literature. Libraries of universities and other institutions typically grant access to a fair number of these databases, through which reviewers can quickly access the literature. PubMed offers free access to all healthcare scientists with online access (National Library of Medicine, National Center for Biotechnology Information, 2021). Although not all articles are freely available via PubMed, the title and abstract can typically be accessed and viewed, so that the reader can ascertain an understanding of the article. In addition to the many databases, there are highly respected and long-established organizations that support the development and housing of rigorously completed literature reviews (e.g., Cochrane, Joanna Briggs Institute, and the Centre for Evidence-Based Medicine) that facilitate further access to information internationally.

The ease of article accessibility seems quite the distance away from a memory of the older of the two authors on this book. She remembers when studying for her dissertation work, she went to the library, checked for potentially relevant articles in large reference books, located the print copy of the articles stored on one of the many rows of large shelves, and printed it on the copier as she methodically inserted coins. Now that very same author (albeit a few years older) can sit down with her cup of tea and her laptop computer and complete an initial advanced search of the literature, download available articles, and order electronic copies by inter-library loan, all in a morning's work. She can also conduct a search of the grey literature on that same laptop, checking on what may have not yet

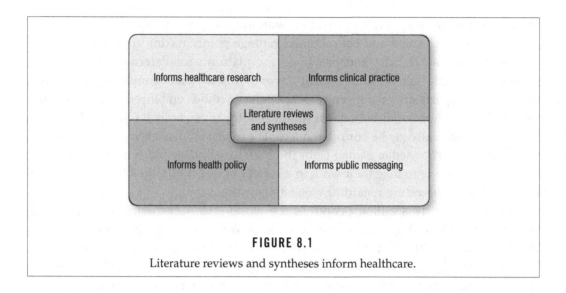

FIGURE 8.1

Literature reviews and syntheses inform healthcare.

made its way to a formal database. However, being able to efficiently and effectively syn-thesize the literature requires the commitment of time, training, and skills, and the ability to locate the resources necessary for appraisal and interpretation (Oh, 2016). These are skills well worth learning and having, as literature reviews and syntheses invaluably con-tribute to understanding and informing healthcare as noted in Figure 8.1. These areas include healthcare research, clinical practice, health policy, and public messaging.

IMPLICATIONS OF LITERATURE REVIEW AND SYNTHESIS ON HEALTHCARE RESEARCH

Literature reviews and syntheses are important to the work of healthcare researchers. Reviews distinctly and comprehensively inform healthcare researchers of the methods, results, and implications of research completed on a given topic to date, as well as an understanding of the research gap. There are many benefits for the reviewer to fully appreciate the research that has and has not been undertaken. Having a solid under-standing of who has conducted which studies, where the studies were conducted, which methods were employed, and key findings provides the reviewer and reader with both an overview and critical specifics about a given topic or question. Repeating studies that have already been conducted which do not require a timely update is not an optimal use of research resources. However, informing research with knowledge generated by prior literature, as well as evidence gaps in a particular context or with specific populations, can be a productive use of a researcher's time.

Awareness of evidence gaps helps to provide specific direction for future research efforts. Reading and understanding the synthesis of the discussion, implications, and future directions of multiple data sources can help determine the magnitude or con-sensus around recommended future research directions. While there is value in recog-nizing what is recommended in peer-reviewed, published literature, we caution that recommendations should be met with a Reviewer's creative innovation. It is useful to appreciate that evidence gaps comprise one aspect of informing future research. The reviewer is advised to combine recommendations for future research with their own expertise, interests, and methodological strengths. The experiences of a reviewer within their role shapes what they determine is necessary and practical for guiding future scholarly endeavors.

We recommend that the reviewer also search the grey literature, including literature with null results. In the event of null findings, it is important for researchers to submit their work for publication, as null findings represent a valuable contribution to the state-of-the-science (Nallamothu et al., 2020). Even if the reviewer can locate null findings in the scientific databases, it is still helpful for the reviewer to examine the grey literature, comprehensively painting a picture of the available evidence on a review topic or question.

IMPLICATIONS OF LITERATURE REVIEW AND SYNTHESIS ON CLINICAL PRACTICE

Healthcare clinicians utilize scientific findings to inform their clinical decision-making, in addition to expert opinion, patient preferences, and other resources. Practice guidelines and recommendations may potentially alter disease trajectory, health outcomes, and, relatedly, quality of life. Furthermore, patient, family, and community preferences, and social and structural determinants of health, will unquestionably shape the decisions regarding one's own health (Eden et al., 2011). Without considering the granularity of the meaning of a literature review to a patient, family, or community, the clinician may lose perspective when studying an area that has the potential to positively contribute at these levels.

The clinician may read the literature review synthesis from several different perspectives, informing how they may approach a patient when discussing the patient's health and healthcare decisions. When a question is sharply focused, a literature review—and most often a systematic review—can provide useful information, including an analysis and interpretation of information that can be used to inform clinical practice (Bolderston, 2008; Cronin et al., 2008). The clinician will assess the possible consequences of a health and healthcare management decision, the potential risks and benefits, and how these considerations are weighed or personalized to each individual patient and/or family. Clinicians may attempt to determine how reliable the evidence is before providing a recommendation. Regarding the evidence, the clinician will want to consider specific features of the patients for whom they are providing care. Literature reviews may provide additional guidance to address those patient-centered considerations (Eden et al., 2011). Examples include age, sex, race and ethnicity, socioeconomic status, or other clinical/diagnostic considerations. For example, with respect to population age, when a clinician is taking care of an infant, the clinician may seek out pediatric-specific literature reviews, in comparison to a healthcare clinician taking care of an individual who is 90 years old, seeking out geriatric-specific literature reviews.

Clinicians often search first for a recent and rigorously completed systematic or other type of literature review on a given topic or question when building upon their current clinical knowledge base. If unable to locate a relevant literature review, they may decide to conduct their own literature review and synthesis (Khan et al., 2011). If time and resources are lacking to conduct their own review, then they may seek out the highest-evidence level of individual studies to inform clinical decision-making.

Systematic reviews have become an integral component of clinical practice guidelines (Moher et al., 2015). When clinical practice guidelines are being created at the regional, national, or international level, it is typical that a comprehensive group of interdisciplinary professionals is gathered. These advisory groups use multiple sources of information to inform their discussion and guideline writing processes, including scientific evidence, their own expert knowledge, and, equally important, the values and preferences of the people whom the guidelines will serve. Scientific evidence includes rigorously completed systematic reviews and meta-analyses. This comprehensive and transparent process informs a solid process for optimizing the quality and outcomes of healthcare provision (Eden et al., 2011; Khan et al., 2011). Clinical practice guidelines help to decrease practice discrepancies and provide standardized guidance for the translation of often complex and vast research into practice settings (Institute of Medicine [IOM], 2011a). Importantly, clinical practice guidelines provide clinicians with the ability to assess benefits and harms in the decision-making process with each individual patient and family.

In contemporary healthcare contexts, clinicians must quickly sort through an expansive body of evidence both for relevancy and quality when making complex clinical decisions (Bettany-Saltikov & McSherry, 2016; Eden et al., 2011). Of particular concern is when evidence is perceived to be biased or non-inclusive of a certain population, rendering it difficult for clinicians to determine how much weight to provide certain evidence. Clinicians should use an objective lens when viewing grey literature that may be industry-sponsored. In rigorous literature reviews and syntheses that include a critical appraisal/quality assessment process, the clinician may be able to use the quality rating to determine the level of the evidence. Critically appraising, assessing the quality, and synthesizing scientific evidence are foundational to clinical practice. As already noted, combining expert information from the literature needs to be coupled with both the judgment of the clinician, as well as the preferences of the patient receiving care (Boland et al., 2017). The increasing demand for evidence-based practice requires an increase in the number of clinicians who have the ability to both generate and synthesize evidence (Oh, 2016).

IMPLICATIONS OF LITERATURE REVIEW AND SYNTHESIS ON HEALTH POLICY

Literature reviews and syntheses are of central importance to health policy processes and decisions, often providing a concise summary of evidence applicable to health policy. For instance, providing information on the effectiveness of an intervention, the outcomes of a program, or an evaluation of the impact of a prior or current policy may serve as the evidence that informs a future health policy decision. When synthesizing the evidence within a literature review, with the professional judgment of a health policy maker, the input of constituents, and resources that are available to enact change, a reviewer can inform important decisions with comprehensive information that has a scientific backing (Boland et al., 2017). Health policy makers may choose to complete a literature review to provide information that will be relevant to a particular policy decision. A concentrated review process can help to address targeted policy questions relatively quickly. As with all literature review teams, health policy decision-makers need to have a team that includes the necessary expertise, skills, and experience to conduct a literature review.

Literature reviews that primarily or secondarily include a cost-effectiveness analysis can guide policy makers in the decision-making process, particularly in a setting with resource constraints (Booth et al., 2016). The actual and projected costs of a program must be informed by not only what the program offers, but also by the anticipated impact, including numbers of persons or communities, as well as predictions of select outcomes. Costs consist of many components, including money, time, and talent, as well as other resources—all of which are finite.

Policy-informing reviews can come in the form of a rapid review, meant to abbreviate the review process timeline to expedite and more quickly inform relevant policy decisions. Reviewers can facilitate the uptake of rapid reviews by developing partnerships with policy makers or health systems managers and providing education about the validity and applicability of rapid review results, as well as how to identify rapid reviews, assess, and interpret findings. While a systematic review is often considered the gold standard to inform a pertinent health policy decision, systematic reviews can be costly regarding time and resources. If there is a short turn-around time available for a health policy decision and a systematic review is not possible, a rapid review may be utilized. However, the reviewer should always follow a rigorous protocol (Grant & Booth, 2009). Early and sustained engagement with the reviewer and the health policy stakeholders are essential for focusing the rapid review and ensuring that it is appropriate to a specific health policy decision of interest. While rapid review methods can be streamlined at many stages of the review process, the review must document and transparently report methodological choices to ensure that the evidence review fits the stated purpose and/or health policy decision. Although rapid reviews can be helpful for healthcare decision-making, policy makers and health systems managers need to consider the context of rapid reviews when using them to inform decision-making. While rapid reviews can inform a busy reader of pertinent issues and considerations, they are necessarily concise (Pautasso, 2013). Rapid reviews are typically shorter in length, and need to be focused to be maximally useful to the policy reader. The rapid review should provide easily and quickly comprehensible study results, emanating from clear and concise methods for reporting statistical analyses. Foci need to be placed on messaging to key audience members, examining results, and detailing policy implications (Tricco et al., 2017).

When rapidly reviewing the literature to inform a policy decision, a reviewer may find evidence risks outweigh any potential benefit. Or there may simply be insufficient evidence available to inform a particular decision. Be aware that actions on the part of individuals or political groups may minimize the findings of a review that offers opposing opinions (Booth et al., 2016). Political interest potentially adds another layer of complexity in the use of literature reviews and syntheses, requiring thoughtful actions by the health policy makers who are working to promote and use science for the betterment of public health.

Having an extensive, methodical review of the literature that is quickly and easily comprehensible is incredibly valuable in health policy realms. A quickly comprehensible review first includes the title and abstract, which is a consolidated overview of the literature review background, methods, results, and conclusions. A short plain-language summary can also provide accurate and easily interpretable information. Executive summaries provide more information than an abstract but are still precisely that: a summary, which should be quick to read and easy for the reader to efficiently comprehend the main points. Executive summaries are designed to display the main points of the literature review within a restricted or abbreviated page count. Further, it is often helpful to display the results of the literature review and synthesis in easily navigable tables. When methodologically appropriate, meta-analyses and meta-syntheses provide concise summarized evidence which can be used to inform policy decision-making. Infographics can be useful as an aesthetically diverse method to convey certain main points or specific sections of a literature review.

IMPLICATIONS OF LITERATURE REVIEW AND SYNTHESIS ON PUBLIC MESSAGING

Literature reviews are undoubtedly instructive in informing healthcare research, clinical practice, and health policy; equally important, however, is ensuring that the public has access and exposure to the knowledge generated by literature reviews in a critical and meaningful way. Researchers and reviewers often publish science in peer-reviewed journals and present at society and other academic conferences. Clinicians contribute to the creation of clinical practice guidelines and are informed by the literature reviews that provide the evidence for evidence-based decisions. Health policy makers leverage literature review approaches to aggregate the literature toward making a health policy decision, which may be implemented at a macro scale. However, when communicating the results of a literature review to the public, different strategies and venues must be considered for maximal public impact.

There is a rapidly expanding number of global media platforms, usable to disseminate the results of a literature review and synthesis to the public. Reviewers have many opportunities to inform the public of their work, such as interviewing with a public news organization, or writing an Op-Ed for a news outlet. Social media, including Twitter, Facebook, and other venues, are platforms that can be used to quickly disseminate literature review work to a large audience. Short video clips on platforms such as YouTube also facilitate the sharing of literature review findings. Additionally, reviewers can create websites or post pertinent information regarding their work on existing websites, such as an institutional research website (in which case the institution's website posting guidelines need to be carefully followed).

Formatting information for the public about your literature review and synthesis requires a distinct and different approach from that used in a peer-reviewed article. How a reviewer formats the findings of their literature review is largely dependent upon the target audience. Using language written at an appropriate literacy level is necessary to effectively deliver your message to the public. We cannot emphasize enough the importance of using language that is tailored to your audience, avoiding jargon and complex sentences. Providing short, succinct messages with key points (e.g., bullets) alongside understandable tables can maximize interpretability and therefore impact. Including a publication date is also important to convey to the reader when the literature review and synthesis was published, as well as including the timeframe of the included data sources. Including pictures, figures, infographics, as well as white space can create a layout that helps the reader more quickly grasp important and key content of the literature review. If needed, the review team can consult with marketing and public relations within their institution for guidance on writing for the public. This can help in ensuring that your messaging retains critical scientific accuracy while appealing to the lay audiences that you are intending to reach.

When you circulate your work in publicly accessible domains, it is essential that you are prepared for the potential positive and negative outcomes that comes with shining a public light on your work. When sharing your work publicly, you may receive interest and praise for your contributions, while still receiving criticism, regardless of your intended impact. This may be particularly true if your literature review and synthesis might reveal controversial findings. For example, your literature review and synthesis may find unexpected and harmful effects of a particular treatment or intervention. If this is the case, you may want to consider working with your public relations, legal team, and/or other experts at your institution to determine how to best convey your literature review and synthesis findings while maintaining strict accuracy on reporting of the results. Know that, in general, if the literature review and synthesis has been carefully and rigorously completed, you can be confident in your synthesis of the findings.

We would be remiss if we did not include a discussion regarding sharing your work with the spoken word, meaning in conversations, for example with your neighbor or someone else with questions whom you might encounter informally. People who are not immersed or familiar with your work may be quite intrigued (or not) with what you are doing and listen attentively (or not). You may encounter disagreement, in which your informal conversational partner may cite a lay article that they read online, a podcast that they recently heard, or a Facebook post that they happened upon which challenges or contradicts your work. This person may also have a relative or friend who had an experience that relates to and potentially challenges your findings. Others may provide examples that are singular and anecdotal and may not necessarily systematically synthesize scientifically derived results. It can be helpful to attempt to understand what is shaping that person's perspective, to listen attentively to any questions, and to assert and respond with objectivity and humility. In these cases, be prepared to provide a respectful, scientifically accurate, understandable, concise, and easily comprehensible response. When the opportunity presents itself, you can explain in lay terms your methods used to derive the review findings, emphasizing the aggregation and synthesis of multiple and rigorously determined scientific sources.

GLOBAL TRENDS IMPACTING LITERATURE REVIEWS AND SYNTHESES

There has been a recent exponential expansion of global access to the internet, diverse new outlets, and social media platforms. Even throughout the writing of this text, the number of media platforms has expanded, as have the options available to display and disseminate information. Media platforms are most relevant and tailored to different audiences, and used in different ways for different purposes by different populations. If in doubt about which media platform to use and how to use it, we recommend that you consult the public relations and/or marketing department at your institution. Always have a solid understanding of the policies that exist pertaining to scientific dissemination within your institution. Also be mindful of a virtual permanence, in that what you post and disseminate is accessible in both real time and for the indefinite future by audiences far and wide. Keep this anticipated permanence front of mind prior to disseminating information on a public media platform, but also do not let this deter scientific dissemination. No healthcare professional wants to see a year, or a decade, or more of work overturned in a moment of misconstrued media attention, while also balancing recognition of the centrality of dissemination to scientific progress.

An increasingly popular trend is that of microlearning. People are consuming and digesting information in partialized units, potentially requiring only 5 to 10 minutes. The trend toward microlearning requires that information be communicated clearly and succinctly. When you are disseminating your literature review findings, it may be surprisingly challenging to determine how to present the information in shorter, consolidated sections. Reviewing the requirements of platforms that you choose to use, and finding examples of similar work can be helpful in making a decision on how to present your work.

There is also the possibility of encountering more publicly challenged or critiqued scholarship. This can present both unique challenges and relatedly, opportunities, for the review team as they interpret, translate, and present their work. This is especially true when evidence on a certain topic or in a particular field is nascent and rapidly evolving as scientists discover more about an issue. A manifestation of this trend has become self-evident in the setting of the COVID-19 pandemic. The collective understanding of the virus and its anticipated global impact change rapidly, as scientists and other healthcare professionals work at lightning speed to understand how to best prevent, diagnose, treat, and vaccinate for the virus. The political climate has also considerably influenced the scientific process and dissemination of related information, undoubtedly influencing public knowledge of the virus.

Evidence and Gap Maps (EGMs) are another tool used to provide guidance on research priorities. While systematic reviews provide a synthesize of the evidence, EGMs provide a summary regarding the availability of evidence and the areas in which the evidence may be sparse or limited. The Campbell Collaboration provides information on developing EGMs (www.campbellcollaboration.org/evidence-gap-maps.html). EGMs are displayed graphically, typically containing a matrix comprised of intervention categories in the rows and the identified outcomes in the columns. EGMs should comply with rules, including following a protocol, a specific established search strategy, specific inclusion and exclusion criteria, and reporting of all studies that meet eligibility criteria. The United Nations Children's Emergency Fund (UNICEF) provides an exemplar for how to create and share EGMs (UNICEF Office of Research—Innocenti, 2021). For specific guidance on EGMs, we refer you to White and colleague's 2020 article on "Guidance for Producing a Campbell Evidence and Gap Map" (www.onlinelibrary.wiley.com/doi/full/10.1002/cl2.1125).

The increasing availability and expanding importance of "big data" also has implications for literature reviews and syntheses, especially on the global scene (Alsunaidi et al., 2021). Researchers can now seek out answers from larger sets of data by analyzing big data sets, as well as conducting meta-analyses (Silva-Fernández & Carmona, 2019). The increasing use of common data elements, minimal data sets, and the same measures across multiple studies, increases the availability of data for researchers to review. These data sets include data points and information on populations that historically would have been difficult to access, now potentially made more easily available for review across borders. This allows for broader comparison, as well as a more nuanced review and understanding of specific populations and issues.

As interest in and the number of literature reviews conducted and published continues to grow, so do the typology of reviews available for reviewers to embark upon. As the number of completed and published literature reviews and syntheses grows, umbrella reviews are becoming increasingly of interest—an option for reviewers when systematic reviews or other types of literature reviews have been completed on a particular topic or question of interest. Mapping reviews serve as another example, aiming to provide a broad overview of individual areas within a certain subject area. By mapping what research has already been completed within a specified area, reading and visualizing this map can provide the reviewer with greater awareness of how to move forward to address a particular gap (Booth et al., 2016). Of note, some types of literature reviews that have not been explored in depth within this text are currently gaining in popularity. For example, desk reviews prompt searching the literature for secondary data sources within a certain area, identify key areas of importance, and apply this information in a reportable format in a subject area, potentially in public health (USAID, 2014). No matter the type of review, the reviewer should understand the methods and approach that provide an unbiased report, adhering to contemporary standards and guidelines for the conduct of the selected type of review.

FINAL THOUGHTS

Providing a conclusion for a book about literature reviews is a bit like fitting a genie in a bottle. There is ample existing information on literature reviews and syntheses, with many experts and organizations leading the way with the conduct and dissemination of exemplary work. To these people that are either working independently or within an organization that provides resources for literature review, we wish to sincerely thank you for taking healthcare science to a level that historically seemed unimaginable. For you, the reviewer, simplistically speaking, there are four key things to remember with your own literature review and synthesis. First, you need to start. Second, you need to work persistently and steadily. Third, you need to finish. Fourth, you need to disseminate your literature review and synthesis contribution to ensure maximal impact. Take time to think about how you will disseminate to the right audiences, and that your literature review and the presentation thereof is sensical and intuitive for your target audience(s). It is also important to keep in mind that literature reviews are a part of the much larger landscape of research and evidence-based practice. Literature reviews and syntheses represent a distinct method poised to provide succinct information that can be used to guide healthcare research, clinical practice, health policy, and public understanding via appropriate messaging. However, literature reviews are still only one component of that process; other scientific evidence, clinical expertise alongside preferences, cultural context, and resources of the people impacted, must also factor strongly into the evidence base and related decisions that directly impact patients, families, and communities. Once you have completed your literature review and synthesis, you will have gained a skill set, and moreover, a way of thinking that will continue to serve you well throughout your career. We encourage you to continue reading literature reviews, periodically update your training in the area of literature reviews and syntheses, commit to finishing the work that you have begun, and always be a critical thinker who is thankful and gracious in the face of the critique that you will receive along the way. We also hope that you celebrate the work that you have done, and recognize and honor the value of the team members that have worked with you to ensure the successful completion of your literature review and synthesis.

ACTIVITIES
Activity I

As a content expert, you have been asked to produce a literature review and synthesis for a report that will be used in a legislative session. You are told that the review must be conducted and the report completed within one month. Fortunately, you are able to clear much of your calendar to engage in this task, as it has been deemed a priority by your institution. Consider how you would answer the following questions.

1. Identify a topic or question on which you identify as an expert.
2. With this topic and question in mind, think about what type of literature review would be a best fit for the topic and objectives, given your one-month timeline.
3. Try to identify potential review team members and justify each of their distinct roles on the team.
4. Create a list of process steps and timeline to follow to complete the literature review by the deadline.
5. Jot down notes on accountability measures to ensure methodological rigor in your review, especially considering the short turnaround time.

Activity II

A recent literature review that you have written has immediate implications for a specific population in your locality. You decide to write an Op-Ed concerning the findings of the review to submit to one of the leading newspapers in your area. Think about how you may approach the Op-Ed writing process, including determining your unique angle. Toward this end, review the following websites for information on writing an Op-Ed. Then, answer the following questions.

www.theopedproject.org/oped-basics

www.commskit.duke.edu/writing-media/writing-effective-op-eds www.nytimes.com/2017 /08/25/opinion/tips-for-aspiring-op-ed-writers.html

1. What are the pros and cons of writing an Op-Ed by yourself or with others? If you decide to write with another person or people, who might you ask to help you to write the Op-Ed?
2. What is your proposed title? Leading line?
3. What elements of your review may be most enticing to highlight?
4. To whom would you alternatively submit your Op-Ed in the event that the intended newspaper decided not to publish it?
5. If you receive a call or message from a colleague or neighbor in response to your Op-Ed, how will you respond to their agreement or disagreement about what you wrote?

SUMMARY POINTS

In this text we have provided for you the necessary steps to conducting your own literature review and synthesis. In this chapter we provide a summary of the reasons justifying the time and cognitive energy investment needed in order to be successful in this work.

- Globally, there are a number of nurses and other healthcare professionals who conduct different types of research. These studies are published in peer-reviewed journals and may be available in the grey literature. This proliferation and availability of literature has in many ways prompted the growing number of literature reviews that are used to guide healthcare research, clinical practice, and health policy, as well as to inform public messaging on a topic.

- Literature reviews and syntheses provide healthcare researchers with rigorous information about work that has already been completed on certain topics, where the evidence gaps exist, as well as implications for future research. Reviewers conduct searches from health-related databases, as well as the grey literature, in order to conduct comprehensive reviews.

- Clinicians use the findings of individual studies and when available, literature reviews, along with their own expertise and patient values and preferences, to make evidence-based clinical decisions. Literature reviews, at a more macro level, are also often used to inform the development and modification of clinical practice guidelines.

When needed, clinicians may also choose to conduct their own literature review and synthesis.

- Health policy decision-makers use literature reviews and syntheses to inform pertinent policy considerations, including cost-effectiveness, as well as risks versus benefits of a particular treatment or intervention. Health policy reviewers may choose to conduct rapid reviews to ensure that science informs policy decisions in a timely manner. Reviewers can also provide executive summaries of their literature reviews for efficient reading and integration into policy decisions.

- The lay public can benefit from literature reviews. Gearing literature review findings toward the public is of the utmost importance, ensuring dissemination and use by diverse audiences. There are several media platforms on which reviewers may choose to share their work. It is important to engage these media platforms wisely to ensure that the message is targeted to the appropriate audience, sometimes verifying regulations and recommendations with a public relations department. It is also advised to engage thoughtfully in conversations with others in a manner that promotes objectivity and humility in conveying literature review findings.

- The exponential expansion of global access to the internet continues to shape the impact of literature reviews. Important trends include microlearning, public challenges of expert recommendations, Evidence and Gap Maps (EGMs), "big data," and the multitude of literature review strategies that continue to influence the conduct and potential of literature reviews and syntheses.

- Exemplary work has been and currently is being completed in the global literature review and synthesis scene. When a reviewer chooses to undertake the literature review process, the reviewer needs to develop a plan to successfully complete the review and disseminate the finished product in a timely manner. Literature reviews are an integral component of the overall database of scientific knowledge that informs healthcare decisions. Once the reviewer has developed the skills to conduct literature reviews, the reviewer has entered into a process where they will continue to learn more over time about literature review and synthesis—an invaluable skill to hold in contributing to the generation of high impact healthcare knowledge.

REFERENCES

Alsunaidi, S. J., Almuhaideb, A. M., Ibrahim, N. M., Shaikh, F. S., Alqudaihi, K. S., Alhaidari, F. A., Khan, I. U., Khan, I. U., Aslam, N., & Alshahrani, M. S. (2021). Applications of big data analytics to control COVID-19 Pandemic. *Sensors, 21*(7), 2282. https://doi.org/10.3390/s2107228

Bettany-Saltikov, J., & McSherry, R. (2016). *How to do a systematic literature review in nursing: A step-by-step guide* (2nd ed.). Open University Press.

Boland, A., Cherry, M. G., & Dickson, R. (2017). *Doing a systematic review: A student's guide* (2nd ed.). Sage.

Bolderston, A. (2008). Writing an effective literature review. *Journal of Medical Imaging and Radiation Sciences, 39*(2), 86–92. https://doi.org/S1939-8654(08)00057-X

Booth, A., Sutton, A., & Papaioannou, D. (2016). *Systematic approaches to a successful literature review* (2nd ed.). SAGE.

Cronin, P., Ryan, F., & Coughlan, M. (2008). Undertaking a literature review: A step-by-step approach. *British Journal of Nursing, 17*(1), 38–43. https://doi.org/10.12968/bjon.2008.17.1.28059

Eden, J., Levit, L., Berg, A., Morton, S., & Committee on Standards for Systematic Reviews of Comparative Effectiveness Research, & Institute of Medicine. (Eds.) (2011). *Finding what works in health care: Standards for systematic review*. The National Academies Press.

Grant, M. J., & Booth, A. (2009). A typology of reviews: An analysis of 14 review types and associated methodologies. *Health Information and Libraries Journal*, *26*(2), 91–108. https://doi.org/10.1111/j.1471-1842.2009.00848.x

Institute of Medicine (US) Committee on Standards for Developing Trustworthy Clinical Practice Guidelines, Graham, R., Mancher, M., Miller Wolman, D., Greenfield, S., & Steinberg, E. (Eds.). (2011). *Clinical practice guidelines we can trust*. National Academies Press.

Khan, K., Kunz, R., Kleijnin, J., & Antes, G. (2011). *Systematic reviews to support evidence-based medicine* (2nd ed.). Hodder Arnold.

Moher, D., Shamseer, L., Clarke, M., Ghersi, D., Liberati, A., Petticrew, M, Shekelle, P., Stewart, L. A., & PRISMA-P Group. (2015). Preferred reporting items for systematic review and meta-analysis protocols (PRISMA-P) 2015 statement. *Systematic Reviews*, *4*, 1-4053-4-1. https://doi.org/10.1186/2046-4053-4-1

Nallamothu, B. K., Schultz, J., & Petty, S. (2020). True negatives: Disseminating research on null, inconclusive, and confirmatory findings in cardiovascular science. *Circulation: Cardiovascular Quality and Outcomes*, *13*(10), 7448. https://doi.org/10.1161/CIRCOUTCOMES.120.007448

National Library of Medicine, National Center for Biotechnology Information. (2021). *Pubmed.gov*. https://pubmed.ncbi.nlm.nih.gov/

Oh, E. G. (2016). Synthesizing quantitative evidence for evidence-based nursing: Systematic review. *Asian Nursing Research*, *10*(2), 89–93. https://doi.org/10.1016/j.anr.2016.05.001

Pautasso, M. (2013). Ten simple rules for writing a literature review. *PLoS Computational Biology*, *9*(7), e1003149. https://doi.org/10.1371/journal.pcbi.1003149

Silva-Fernández, L., & Carmona, L. (2019). Meta-analysis in the era of big data. *Clinical Rheumatology*, *38*, 2027–2028. https://doi.org/10.1007/s10067-019-04666-3

Tricco, A. C., Langlois, E. V., & Straus, S. E. (Eds.) (2017). *Rapid reviews to strengthen health policy and systems: A practical guide*. World Health Organization. https://apps.who.int/iris/bitstream/handle/10665/258698/9789241512763-eng.pdf;jsessionid=9A9AED7961D0D17D819AF294F5B96218?sequence=1

UNICEF Office of Research - Innocenti. (2021). *Evidence gap maps*. https://www.unicef-irc.org/evidence-gap-maps

United States Census Bureau. (2021). *U.S. and world population clock*. https://www.census.gov/popclock/world

USAID. (2014). *Step 1: Complete desk review*. https://assessment-action.net/wp-content/uploads/2014/03/Phase-2-LEARN-Overview.pdf

Index

Printed in the United States
by Baker & Taylor Publisher Services